A SMELL
OF BURNING

A SMELL
OF BURNING

THE STORY OF
EPILEPSY

Colin Grant

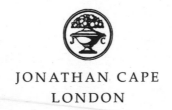

JONATHAN CAPE
LONDON

1 3 5 7 9 10 8 6 4 2

Jonathan Cape, an imprint of Vintage Publishing,
20 Vauxhall Bridge Road,
London SW1V 2SA

Jonathan Cape is part of the Penguin Random House group of companies whose
addresses can be found at global.penguinrandomhouse.com

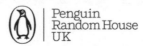

Penguin
Random House
UK

Copyright © Colin Grant 2016

First published by Jonathan Cape in 2016

penguin.co.uk/vintage

A CIP catalogue record for this book is available from the British Library

Hardback ISBN 9780224101820

Typeset in Adobe Caslon by Thomson Digital Pvt Ltd, Noida, Delhi

Printed and bound in Great Britain by Clays Ltd, St Ives PLC

Penguin Random House is committed to a sustainable future
for our business, our readers and our planet. This book is made
from Forest Stewardship Council® certified paper.

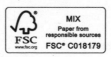

MIX
Paper from
responsible sources
FSC® C018179

Contents

Preface

'Are you epileptic?' Almost everyone asked this when I told them that I was writing a book on epilepsy. I would like to have said 'yes' to see where the conversation went. On some level, answering 'no' felt like a betrayal. When they followed up with the question, 'Why are you writing about it?' I would describe a scenario:

A man writhes on the ground. His arms slap and snap about him. His legs kick out at some invisible enemy. His head twists from side to side. A strange guttural sound comes from his throat and his mouth froths with foam. Your journey to work is abruptly interrupted by the sight of him. Perhaps the man is drunk. Could he be having a fit? You've heard of such a thing but doubt whether you've ever seen one. Then again, maybe he is just drunk. Yes, he probably brought it on himself. In any event you calculate that this is something you cannot deal with. You are paralysed with indecision and look about you. Another person will pass by soon. You move on. Of course you do.

You get to work and play back the incident in your head. A sense of guilt courses through your body as you admit to yourself that obviously you knew what it was all along. 'That man,' I would tell the people who asked about the book, 'is my brother, Christopher.'

The man suffers from epilepsy, a word derived from the Greek for 'to capture' or 'to seize', which describes perfectly how the disease temporarily takes hold of a person. The seizures are a manifestation of a spooky condition – ancient, shadowy and violent – for which there is no known cure. But why, after a thoroughly modern education and earnest campaigns of demystification, are we still fearful of people with epilepsy; and why are they so ashamed of their condition?

The uncontrolled spasms seem so bizarre and terrifying to the beholder that for much of human history people with epilepsy were thought to be possessed by devils. Not until the nineteenth century did we get a clearer picture of what was going on, when the pioneering neurologist, John Hughlings Jackson, defined an epileptic seizure as 'an occasional sudden excessive, rapid and local discharge in the grey matter [of the brain]'.[1] It is now possible to imagine a storm of electrical interference that disrupts normal brain function. Only that is on the inside. When a person with epilepsy has a fit what we see on the outside is his sudden frailty, and his pitiful body wracked by an inexplicable paroxysm.

Through decades of discussion, reportage and advances in treatment, our anxieties over cancer and other potentially life-threatening diseases have diminished. Cancer is no longer a whispered 'fear word'. The same is not true for epilepsy. Our response to it defies rationality. Why, more than in other conditions, does our dealing with epilepsy remain almost primal? Why, when the centuries-old link between epilepsy and mental ill health has finally been broken, do we quietly reassemble it in our heads when observing a man having a fit in the street?

For much of history only one form of seizure, the graphic grand mal, was ever recognised. But in the last century, scientists have been able to finesse the broad brushstrokes of our ancestors' descriptions of epilepsy to discern numerous forms. Epilepsy, then, is an umbrella term under which seizures fall. Still, there are two main categories: generalised seizures, in both hemispheres of the brain, for which there is no known cause (though inheritance is considered a factor in many cases); and focal or partial seizures which arise in a particular damaged or sensitised part of the brain as a result of congenital disease or trauma, such as a blow to the head.

The story of epilepsy is a remarkable one. If it's a shameful, brutal and bruising tale it is also one of redemption. People with epilepsy have resisted and survived purges and pathological attempts to eradicate them as if they were defective carriers of a contagious disease. Throughout history marriage of epileptics was discouraged, and their castration has been strongly proposed to rid humanity of their affliction. In the 1930s and 1940s, under the Nazi eugenics programme, the forced sterilisation of epileptics reached its apogee. But one of the greatest confounders or disrupters to this narrative has been the fact of the large number of famous people known or suspected to have been epileptic. They include Julius Caesar, Joan of Arc, Fyodor Dostoevsky, Edward Lear, Vincent Van Gogh, Harriet Tubman, Vladimir Ilich Lenin, Neil Young and many more.

For some the association with the likes of Caesar lends the condition a kind of glamour, carrying with it the suggestion that it is a disease of the great; for others the fear and awe felt about it is most marked in the crossover between epilepsy and religion as recorded for instance in the visions of Joan of Arc.

In our secular age, scientific inquiry into the relationship between extrasensory perception and temporal lobe epilepsy highlights neurological connections rather than spiritual ones. We look more closely at the fact that in the mind of the nineteenth-century abolitionist, Harriet Tubman, God's voice and her visions of Zion grew more strongly after she was struck on the head by her slave owner with a heavy metal bar.

No matter the cause, the onset of epilepsy is a puzzle. The condition lies dormant until it is first triggered and then there's no going back. The initial fit will inevitably result in subsequent fits; so that, as the neurologist William Gowers once suggested, 'every fit may be said to be the result of those which have preceded it, and the cause of those that follow it'.[2] But the initial stimulus for the fit, Gowers noted, 'bears no more causal relation to the disease than does a spark to the explosion of the gun powder on which it falls'. The real cause lies within the brain, and remains unknown.

The severity of generalised seizures ranges from minor to major electrical disturbances of the brain; from petit mal where the person with epilepsy suffers minor, mostly unnoticeable absences (gone in a blink), to the grand mal major seizures in which the whole body suffers violent convulsions. The real paradox is that epileptic seizures are rarely witnessed yet are extremely common. There are more than 60 million sufferers on the planet. More than half of all cases are diagnosed before the age of twenty-five. That was certainly true of Christopher.

In the years that followed his diagnosis, we settled into a ritual during and after each seizure. I would lean over him, ensuring that his tongue was freed from his clenched teeth, and wait and pray for his eyes to open. I often wondered where Christopher went in those moments. Sometimes I imagined him in a kind of netherworld, like David Niven in the film *A Matter of Life and Death*, negotiating with God's foppish Napoleonic emissary. Despite the clinical explanations, epilepsy seemed a mystery to me: it was ghostly, otherworldly and uncanny.

It is often assumed that epilepsy is a rare condition, but consistently it affects one per cent of the world's population from Delaware to Delhi. Every carriage of every commuter train is likely to have a person with epilepsy on board. But if, as is probable, there's someone in your office who's prone to fits, he's unlikely to be shouting about it. Many people with epilepsy still live in fear of exposure.

If you imagined the history of epilepsy contained in one person, a several-thousand-year-old man perhaps, what tale would he tell?

Let's say he was born in ancient Sparta. Then, as a baby, he was washed in wine to see whether he convulsed. He did, but instead of being abandoned and left to die, somehow he survived.

Later, he was sold as a slave. But the ancient Hammurabi code stipulated that a slave could be returned and a demand made for the money to be refunded, if *bennu* (epilepsy) appeared within the month after the purchase. He was returned as worthless.

Our epileptic everyman became a legionary in the Roman army and swears he saw Caesar fall down at the Battle of Thapsus with an affliction akin to his own, but that he never spoke of it.

In the Middle Ages he was called a warlock and threatened to be burned at the stake. He's been locked up in asylums and put on display at a kind of freak show run by neurologists in Paris. Rarely has he worked, but his employment prospects improved when he found refuge in a nineteenth-century epileptics' colony.

He's had his share of medical interventions. Bromide didn't help, nor trephination, nor temporal lobectomy. He has lived fearfully in epilepsy's shadow. Always the pattern is the same: the paroxysm threatens to arrive, makes itself known and then disappears. Mercifully, he does not remember the actual fits. But there are sensations that have haunted him all his life: the detritus of seizures; and, worse still, the acrid odour of foreboding that announces each new fit. His prognosis is poor and there is no end in sight.

Despite the reflected glamour of some of those associated with the disease, epilepsy is still mysterious, an enigma and something of a taboo subject. We may have conquered our fear of carcinomas but conditions like epilepsy remain truly disturbing.

The story of epilepsy is a tale of fear and loathing, and seemingly intractable ignorance; of humane neurologists; of a pioneering brain surgeon who desired to alleviate the suffering of his son; of the afflicted starting new lives in epileptic colonies in Germany, Britain and the USA; of one Russian, Fyodor Dostoevsky, who converted his epilepsy into art, and of another, Vladimir Ilich Lenin, who died from a prolonged seizure – in *status epilepticus*. It's also my brother's tale.

People with epilepsy lead parallel lives to most of mainstream society. Some of us will have gained insights into those lives through a handful of literary works, or seen tender studies of epileptics in the atlas of Esquirol's *Des Maladies Mentales*. But the closest most of us will get to a person with epilepsy is when we sit down in the cinema and observe the graphic depiction of convulsions on screen, in ways that render the individual invisible. Christopher's story, as well as that of many other sufferers down the years, offers a window into the world of epilepsy.

The story of epilepsy zigzags through history. The chronology is never straightforward. At times it appears that ancient Greece had a far more sophisticated approach to the condition than medieval Europe. A study of the condition lets us into the beauty of the physiology of the brain and offers tantalising glimpses into how consciousness might be formed in the white and grey matter. It also introduces us to the torment of living on amber alert, and the impact of this aberrant electrical activity on a life lived in fear; of not knowing when an attack will happen; of mental absences; of loss of memory and control.

Epilepsy has many negative associations. But if, as I believe, there are aspects of the disease that can be described as positive phenomena, then in the ledger of epilepsy where do the credits and deficits fall?

Some people with epilepsy are concerned about the way that severe grand mal seizures result in a certain dulling of the senses and a fear of declining mental ability. But did temporal-lobe seizures diminish or explode the mental capacity of Joan of Arc? Had it not been for her seizures, would Harriet Tubman have been quite as brave? At the height of the Atlantic slave trade, did visions uncouple a rational freight of fear of a recently freed woman allowing her to return again and again to the treacherous American South to lead others like her out of captivity?

Science stands accused regularly of cold-hearted revisionism. But a bigger complaint is that too many overly optimistic claims are made for neuroscience that cannot be supported. Advances in neural imaging have given scientists a greater understanding of the electrical disturbances that occur in the brain during seizures. But for sufferers of intractable epilepsy, is the last-ditch surgical option of removing slivers of damaged brain tissue little more attractive than the first fumbling of the split-brain operations of the early 1960s? Advances in the treatment of epilepsy have been contingent on our greater understanding of neurology; but then that sentence could be reversed. If neurology is the chicken then epilepsy is the egg. John Hughlings Jackson, a pioneer in neurology, put it succinctly: 'He who is faithfully analysing many different cases of epilepsy is doing far more than studying epilepsy. The highest centres, those concerned in such fits, represent all, literally all, parts of the body sensorily and motorily, in most complex ways, in most intricate combinations, etc.'[3] A close study of epileptic fits has thus been key to illuminating the workings of the 'organ of the mind'; and for that we are indebted to people with epilepsy – those who were subject to experimental investigations and treatments, voluntarily and involuntarily.

Just Awake

The patient was not inviting. Though he did not stir as I approached, I sensed some part of him turn away. He lay on top of the undisturbed bed sheets, arched, with his hands behind his head as if in a hammock, staring up towards the ceiling at nothing in particular.

Barely a third of the way through the ward round, I had been dispatched by the consultant to 'be so good' as to go to the adjoining ward and take this man's medical history. At this stage of my career taking a history was still something of a novelty. It was only my third time, and a challenge that always induced a sense of urgency, as if I was a participant in the TV game show *It's a Knockout*. I had approximately thirty minutes before the consultant (a strutting, imperious peacock) and his remaining retinue (his train of peacock feathers) caught up with me. The patient was to be the subject of my first-ever ward round presentation.

Boredom could not explain his languor. Only reluctantly did he move his feet, as I felt for somewhere to sit at the edge of his bed. I suspect that every student, like me, had entered medical school with an expectation of reverence and gratitude on the part of patients, yet the sick man in front of me exuded a kind of resentment.

In our introductory years we had been kept away from real live patients. The only patients we initially encountered were dead; we spent a year dissecting them. According to the eighteenth-century

surgeon William Hunter, dissection toughened up students and
prospective surgeons as 'it informs the head, guides the hand,
and familiarizes the heart to a kind of necessary inhumanity'.[1]
Dissection afforded us the luxury of learning anatomy from patients
who couldn't scream when their hearts were removed and their
skulls were sawn in two. But the hands-on experience with a corpse
also gave the fledgling student a chance to come to terms with
his natural discomfort over what was to become a lifetime of
enforced familiarity with strangers. The dead were proxy for the
living. Though cutting up a cadaver wouldn't necessarily prepare
us for the future embarrassment, for example, of rectal examinations,
it might take us part of the way.

In medicine to 'take a history' is to embark on the first inves-
tigative step towards diagnosis. The mantra, drilled into every
student, is that the answer to your patient's present condition lies
in the past. Thirty years ago, at the London Hospital, it was soon
apparent that taking a history was what I enjoyed most, even
though (and perhaps because) the process was so maddening, with
patients often starting in the middle of the story, lurching forward
to the present and then shuttling back to the past.

In that summer of 1984, as I perched on the edge of the hospital
bed in that general ward, in my freshly starched white coat and
with a stethoscope draped over my shoulders (rather glamorously
actually), I immediately started looking for clues. Elbowing his
way up the bed, the forty-something-year-old patient in front of
me struggled to sit up straight, and refused to answer my smile.
He had the countenance of someone who'd weathered a thousand
tiny insults; they were etched into the lines of his forehead and
cheeks. He had the drawn, inelastic face of either a serious smoker
(with no time for the inconvenience of food) or a fastidious vegan
whose pursuit of a healthy lifestyle had left him on the verge of
sickness.

I opened my A4 folder and turned to the first clean sheet, pen poised. 'So what appears to be the problem? Why are you here?' I asked.

Nothing. He looked straight ahead but his eyes did not or could not focus on me. It was as if he were on the mirrored side of a two-way mirror. I could inspect him up close but he appeared not to see me. For a moment I suspected that he was blind, but he blinked when I waved a finger in front of him.

On the long, high-ceilinged ward, the constant drone of the floor-polishing machine camouflaged conversations. So that even though it was an open ward, with no screens to soften sound, taking a history could be conducted with a degree of confessional privacy.

I tried again. 'So can you tell me why you're here?'

'Just awake,' he whispered.

'Do you know where you are?'

'Just awake,' he answered more forcefully than before.

'How about the year? What year is it?'

He appeared to sigh, 'Just awake.'

'Can you tell me the name of the king or queen?' I asked. 'Who is the monarch on the throne?'

'Just awake!'

'Just awake?' I left a gap for him to complete the sentence or thought.

'Just awake.'

And so it went on. His truculence – if that's what it was – was unnerving. It mocked my white coat and stethoscope, my playing at being a doctor. And after yet another dismissive 'Just awake' the dread of being found out – the fear every medical student constantly carries around of being unmasked as an incompetent – crept into my voice. I ploughed on unthinkingly through the questionnaire, barely resisting the idea that I should somehow steal away from the patient before the ward round reached his bed. I pictured having to read back his sparse medical history to the consultant who, I noticed, had just entered the ward. There were perhaps a dozen beds between us but the ward round was inexorably wending its way towards me.

'Be so good,' the consultant had said. He'd made it sound as though I was doing him a favour; but I was under no illusions as to what was in store. We, the students, were the meat; the consultant was the skewer. By our third year, we all understood that, despite the occasional nod towards new-fangled ideas such as 'role playing', our medical education was predicated on a tradition of ritualistic humiliation.

But then on the twelfth or thirteenth 'Just awake', it dawned on me that this was, in fact, all the patient could say. Through some bizarre neurological accident his vocabulary had become limited to these two words. From then on we worked out a code: I'd ask a question, such as, 'Has this happened before?' And he'd reply, 'Just awake.' But, through his drawl, inflection, emphasis or tone, I could infer his intended response. We had a conversation. I gleaned that he had had a seizure; that he could remember where he was before the epileptic attack (placing a bet at Ladbrokes on Whitechapel High Street), but that he had no recollection of anything thereafter. When he had roused himself from the fit he was 'Just awake'.

I know now that he was also suffering from a temporary aphasia following the seizure; that he was only capable of a few words of 'telegraphic speech' or 'emotional ejaculation'. After fifteen minutes of inquisition the patient started to tire. With each subsequent question he slipped further and further down the bed. So that, towards the end of my history-taking, he was virtually horizontal. I felt a little like a guest who had outstayed his welcome and began to make my apologies and to thank him for his time.

It was then that I noticed the strange gurgling sounds coming from the patient, and the spasms like someone with particularly violent hiccups. His legs and torso rose slightly from the bed and then he began to shake.

'Nurse, nurse,' I cried.

Some medics immediately peeled away from the outer fringes of the ward round. They descended on us as spectacularly as a crash team. Their urgent but precise movements had the quality of rehearsed choreography; a silver trolley on wheels arrived from nowhere; plastic gloves were snapped on. More and more doctors and nurses began to arrive; so many in fact that I was brushed aside as the grey curtain in one continuous action was pulled around the backs of the medics to enclose the bed. When it was fully closed I found myself on the wrong side of the curtains, on the outside. I could hear, though, the quick decisions being made; and soon after a suppository was administered, the patient stopped shaking. The consultant arrived. He had a self-regarding tempo, markedly different from everyone else. He moved purposefully but not in a hurry. After all, there was no emergency that couldn't wait.

He pulled back the curtain as a star might on making his entrance to the stage. The staff froze momentarily until the consultant, taking in all that was unfolding, nodded for them to continue. The team parted to make room for him and the curtain swished back closed.

'What's his medication?' asked the consultant.

'We think he's non-compliant,' someone answered.

'Is?' said the consultant incredulously. '*Is* non-compliant?'

'Yes, is.'

'You mean was, surely. He was non-compliant. He doesn't have much choice now, does he? Not now you've shoved a bloody suppository up his arse.'

There was silence whilst the team seemed to weigh whether the consultant had made a joke or not. It might conceivably be an admonition.

'What about the history?' said the consultant angrily. 'Who's taken the history?'

There was another silence – this time, though, not a complete one; it was punctuated by a few nervous coughs and splutters like the hubbub of an expectant audience just before the orchestra launches into the first piece. I backed away, still facing the direction of the curtained-off bed lest my absence was suddenly realised; and as I departed through the swing doors I could hear the muffled sound of the consultant barking.

My failed presentation had been an introduction to the dictatorship of the hospital ward, and to the drama and indignities of epilepsy. When the patient did awake he would find himself being prodded and scrutinised by half a dozen medics. I had thought that the curtains had been drawn out of respect for him and the preservation of his dignity. But what about the humiliation of waking to a set of strangers who had borne witness to a very public display of your private anguish? And now it seemed that far from sparing the epileptic, the curtains had been drawn to spare the neighbouring patients the sight of someone having a fit.

And he need not have had a seizure – so I thought then – if I had made the diagnosis quicker. In *The Idiot*, Fyodor Dostoevsky writes of his epileptic protagonist, Prince Myshkin, that you'd be able to guess straight away that he was epileptic.[2] Dostoevsky, who suffered from the condition from childhood, was better placed than most to detect the condition in others. But is it possible to pick an epileptic out of a crowd?

In the days that followed the ward round, I began to feel that I had failed the patient; that I had recoiled from him and called for help, as a lay person might, out of shock at the spectacle of his seizure. I could not conceive of a follow-up session with him, completing his medical history. I imagined that he would have felt violated and horribly exposed when he woke up; and by now he'd be conscious of the fact that I, too, had been present during his fit. Still, I was intrigued by him, by his frailty and by my own sense of guilt at being a young adult hungry for novel and heightened experiences. For it had to be admitted that, as well as repulsion, there was a prurient fascination in witnessing the otherworldliness of someone in the grip of a grand mal seizure.

And then something worse emerged. An unwelcome thought started to develop in the forefront of my brain: what if he hadn't woken up? I was not present when the patient had revived. What if he hadn't fully regained consciousness? It was rare for people to die during a fit but it was not unknown. Lenin, I'd learnt only recently, had suffered *status epilepticus*, an unbroken seizure that went on for forty-five minutes, before his death.

Even in the midst of these fragile thoughts, I upbraided myself for being so foolish. Wasn't that why they gave my patient a suppository (a muscle relaxant to break the spasms of the fit) in the first place? But then why all the excitement if the medical intervention only amounted to administering a suppository? And why the mad barking by the consultant at the end?

For a whole day and night I was plagued by the notion of a negative outcome; that something had gone terribly wrong with the epileptic patient. I hadn't even found out what he was called; and I never did, because when I returned eventually, out of a sense of duty and of atonement, to that ward, he was nowhere to be seen. Another patient was occupying his bed, and I was too afraid to enquire of the nursing staff what had become of the man who was 'Just awake'.

The encounter with that patient was my first with epilepsy; but it was not to be the last. Over the coming years, mental absences, petit mal and grand mal seizures, and the full spectrum of epileptic attacks, were to feature regularly in my life.

The first time that my teenage brother, Christopher, failed to emerge from the bathroom and we had to break down the door to free him, we dismissed the fainting incident as bizarre but amusing. By the third occasion, following a battery of tests including a fitful night at a sleep-deprivation clinic, I began to entertain the alarming suspicion that the fainting episodes were really epileptic seizures.

I was as reticent as my brother in entertaining such an unwanted diagnosis. It seemed most improbable and terrifying. To accept such a diagnosis was to surrender to a new set of unexpected limits on your life (as I imagined that first patient had); to let go of all of your dreams and aspirations; and to sign up to an extraordinary transformation that not even Hollywood in its wildest and most ludicrous fantasies was capable of.

Best Kept Secret

Even though we were in the kitchen, at the back of the house, the drone from the M1 motorway, perhaps half a mile away, was immense.

'Is it always this noisy?' I asked my mother.

'You hear something?'

'No, it doesn't matter. I was just saying.'

I'd left home four years earlier and it was strange to think that throughout my childhood in Farley Hill that background hum of speeding cars on asphalt, fenced off from the estate, had always been there but that I'd never noticed until now.

My mum returned to the theme of the night; to the reason why I'd been summoned from medical school in London to our home in Luton, to the kitchen where we'd sat from the early evening till now close to midnight (so absorbed that as dusk had fallen we had forgotten to switch on the overhead ceiling light) with my mother drawing up an inventory of her problems.

Christopher, at fifteen her youngest child, had had two more collapses since the first a month ago. 'I grow to hate that sound, you see,' she said of the awful thud of his body hitting the ground. We talked through the night, with the moonlight throwing shadows across the walls and kitchen table; there was really only one subject. I liked the intimacy of the dark. It made it easier to talk.

'How can he be all right one minute, and then this?'

'Christopher?'

'Yes. You never see anything?'

For as long as I could remember I'd been charged with watching over my baby brother. Christopher occupied a unique position in our family. He was the youngest, the most exuberant and happy. He seemed a blessed being who gladdened the heart of even the most miserable. It was as if, miraculously, his card had not been marked. At home, our tyrannical father Bageye threatened always to explode, but in the presence of Christopher he was disarmed.

After separating from Bageye, our mother had brought up seven children on her own. She'd been constantly on the move: rushing to the town hall to pay the rent; taking on overtime at Vauxhall Motors; popping over to the neighbours to borrow just enough to ward off the bailiffs. Throughout the 1970s, 'soon come' was our mother's watchword. She would soon come from whatever emergency she'd have to fix before it was succeeded by the next one; and in the meantime, could I keep an eye on my baby brother? It wasn't too much to ask, surely. But lately it was a role I hadn't been able to sustain as a student at the London Hospital; and Christopher's recent fainting episodes had taken her back to that decades-old daily anxiety. It had alarmed her so much, she'd sent for me for reassurance.

'Something is wrong.' Her heavy words barely supported a horrible truth that was going to come crashing down. 'Evil must have come into the house.'

She meant the evil that had befallen Christopher.

'I don't think it's the devil's work. Come on now, Mum, it's not the devil. You don't really believe that. It's something else.'

'Tell me, then. I must know. You can tell me, you know.'

I hesitated. 'I'm not sure.'

'You just there humouring me,' she said gravely. 'I carry you for nine months. I must know when my child is bluffing.'

'Well, it's, you know, it's epilepsy, isn't it? Don't you think?'

'Yes, Lord,' she cried out immediately. 'Anybody see my cross? Anybody see my cross?' She had suspected it all along but now I'd said it, the great flood of emotion burst through her chest. She heaved. She breathed heavily, howling and wailing, 'Yes, Lord, Yes, Lord.'

I could find no words to console her. I sat in silence, cowardly, averting my gaze. After some time the sobbing subsided and was driven out and replaced by the unremitting drone of the f'ing motorway.

'Oh, I hear it now,' she whispered, drying her eyes.

I placed a hand on her arm and slowly, snivelling, she composed herself. 'Don't tell him a thing.'

'Who? Christopher?'

'Don't tell him a thing. Promise me. I beg you.'

In 1926, Graham Greene was summoned by his doctor to alert him to a serious condition that carried certain risks which he must 'consider carefully before marriage'. The diagnosis had already been given to his parents some months earlier, after Greene suffered a bout of fainting, but it had been agreed that the secret was best kept from their son; that he 'ought not to be told what the matter is in any terms that included the word epilepsy'.

Writing in his autobiography, *A Sort of Life*, Graham Greene recalled that at that time epilepsy ranked alongside cancer and leprosy as the condition most feared by the British public. Even though Greene's physician held out the hope that his epileptic episodes might be arrested by 'good walks and Kepler's Malt Extract', the fledgling, twenty-two-year-old writer was devastated. He'd recently pledged himself to be married, but now he was being counselled about the risks of fatherhood as epilepsy could be inherited. The next day Graham Greene found himself 'standing on an Underground platform . . . trying to summon the will and courage to jump'.[1]

Ancient Romans believed that sex might prevent epilepsy, but other cultures before and after contended that the opposite was true. In England the prevailing view of epilepsy and marriage had not much changed from when the Victorian physician Sir Edward Sieveking wrote in his study *On Epilepsy* in 1857, '[T]he marital act itself may become an exciting cause of epilepsy, and as we know the hereditary influence of the disease is great, we ought not to counsel epileptics to marry.'[2]

Greene confided that in contemplating suicide, he was exhausted 'by the thought of starting a completely different future' from the one he'd imagined for himself. Paralysed with indecision on the Underground platform, Greene recalled, 'the trains came and went, and soon I took the moving staircase to the upper world'. But his despair was not at an end. Graham Greene's recent conversion to Catholicism presented a further ethical complication. In the event of marriage, contraception would not be countenanced and the possibility of passing on the condition to his children was very real. He sought counsel from an elderly priest, but there was no solace, just a pedantic line of argument that was a 'useless embroidery that made no pattern'.[3] In the event, his conscience was not tested. Greene's questioning of, and doubt over, the diagnosis was supported by his brother who was a doctor. Luckily, for some people with epilepsy, their seizures are finite: they come to an end without medical intervention but although there would be no further fainting attacks, he had been given a significant jolt.

Class had a bearing on the stigma of epilepsy in British society at the time. The neurologist William Gowers observed that the middle and upper classes were much more disinclined than the working class to admit to epilepsy in their families or circle of friends. Perhaps those lower down the social ladder did not have so much to lose; epilepsy was just one more stigma to add to their lot.[4]

Graham Greene later confronted his parents over their tardiness in informing him about their suspicions, but he sympathised with their plight; any criticism of them was tempered by the knowledge of their intent to shield him from the frightening revelation of epilepsy and the subsequent negative impact it might have had on his future.

In Britain, up until 1970, when at the climax of the marriage ceremony the priest asks the witnesses whether they know of any reason why the couple before them should not be wedded, the answer would be 'yes' if bride or groom were known to be epileptic. Under the Matrimonial Causes Act 1937, a marriage could be made void if 'either party was, at the time of marriage, of unsound mind, mentally defective or subject to recurrent fits of insanity or epilepsy'. That law was repealed in Britain in 1970, and similarly the year earlier in Finland, but comparable legislation was still being enforced around the globe.

Epilepsy is considered by the courts of numerous countries including Kenya, Jamaica and Nigeria to be grounds for a decree of nullity of marriage. And it is still the subject of legal challenges in many parts of the world, most notably India. Under the Hindu Marriage Act of 1955, a wedding could only be solemnised 'if at the time of marriage neither party suffers from recurrent attacks of insanity or epilepsy'. Though this proviso was amended in 1999 so that the words 'or epilepsy' were omitted, plaintiffs regularly petition the courts for divorce on matrimonial grounds of 'unsoundness of mind' or 'epileptic insanity'. Fraud is also often cited as a reason for nullifying the marriage where a plaintiff suggests that the spouse knew of their epilepsy but failed to disclose the condition. In 2007, a survey amongst women attending an epilepsy clinic in Kerala found that a majority concealed their epilepsy from their prospective spouse at the time of marriage, and that they did so largely because they feared disclosure would lead to a breakdown of marriage negotiations.

*

I interviewed a number of people with epilepsy for this book, including Sian who had been married to Malik. People were always struck by Malik. Because he was said to come from Saudi Arabia, he soon acquired the nickname 'Wallet'. It suited his largesse. He was especially generous towards Sian, with whom he appeared smitten. After university, Sian told me, it seemed inevitable that they would marry, but in the event, they could not wait till their final year. Sian became pregnant and that settled the matter. Though she sometimes struggled to read him through his hooded eyes, he was ever watchful of her. She was especially touched by his attentiveness to the discomforts of pregnancy; more phlegmatic than tender perhaps, but she preferred it that way.

The only extensive disagreement they had was over the prospective name for their child. It lasted a week. At first he had argued reasonably. Then at the end of the week, he simply announced, 'A decision has been reached. Naghib.' When she asked why he was so determined, he simply answered that it was a good Egyptian name.

Sian was taken aback. Like everyone, she'd thought him a Saudi. True, he hadn't volunteered that information but equally he'd never contradicted her. In the end, neither had their way over the child's name because three months later Sian miscarried.

In the days leading up to graduation, Malik announced that he'd been offered a family job back in Alexandria and that the newlyweds would be setting up home there. Within weeks of the return the marriage started to unravel. Though they'd never really discussed her condition, Sian located the root of the trouble in her epilepsy; in particular to the occasion when a seizure was witnessed by Malik's mother and siblings. Sian noted a sudden cooling of her relationship with Malik. They no longer slept together, after Malik, scouring the Internet, stumbled across a chat room that suggested that intimacy brought on fits.

And then one day something unfathomable happened: Malik beat Sian. That seemed to release something in him. He beat her following each subsequent epileptic attack; and she realised that he was somehow trying to exorcise the seizures. Sian had brought shame on him *and* his family. He solicited a lawyer to petition the courts; he would sue for divorce on the grounds that she had hidden her epileptic condition from him. And Malik raised no objection when Sian wrote to her brother to ask for his help in bringing her back to the UK.

The year before, prior to setting out for Alexandria with her husband, Sian had been tormented by the idea that her colour or culture might prove problematic for Malik's family; she had never imagined the possibility that her marriage could founder as a result of prejudices around epilepsy.[5]

The notion of shame and the maxim 'Death before dishonour' must have infected me as a child. Its power came from the fact of it being Bageye's phrase – one of the few things he ever said and yet he voiced it so often that it became a mantra. It had a rigid Old Testament profundity that suited his character. The consequences of any breach of this golden rule, of your dishonourable conduct being brought to his attention, were too terrifying to contemplate. I imagined the saying as a giant belt that girded our house on Farley Hill. And somehow the latent terror Bageye instilled outlasted his presence in the household.

I suppose from the age of about thirteen I had been a father to my brother, after Bageye was shown the front door and discouraged from ever returning. In the days following Christopher's first fainting fit in the bathroom, I was tormented by a kind of déjà vu; that I had witnessed in my brother earlier signs of what must have been epilepsy. Though until summoned by my mother I had kept my own counsel, trawling through my remembrance of

Christopher's childhood now I recalled an unsettling incident at our local Catholic church six or seven years earlier when he'd apparently fainted.

That dormant memory was discoloured by my antipathy towards the priest into whose malign realm I had unthinkingly delivered my brother as an altar boy when he was seven. The priest was no good. He found everybody in the congregation disagreeable apart from the biggest donors to the collection plate and the women who cleaned and cooked for him. He held disgust in his nose, a magnificent, diaphanous beak with thread-like blue veins and tobacco stains on the nostril hair and dividing septum, usually slightly cocked and in a permanent sneer.

In the beginning, I'd been charmed by the possibilities of beatification that service as an altar boy seemed to offer; and when Christopher's turn came to kneel at the altar, though he did not say as much, I imagine he felt it too. I would not have wanted to sully his innocent expectation with my cynicism. I left and he joined the ranks of altar boys; a world where humility could not save you from humiliation; where guilt and shame were hardly leavened by innocence.

Nonetheless, being an altar boy marked you out, especially so on important ceremonies such as the 'washing of the feet' when Father Monroe played the humble Christ and the boys his unworthy apostles in a re-enactment of the Last Supper. The boys had drawn lots as to which apostle they'd represent in the ceremony. Christopher wouldn't say whom he'd been given but as the day grew closer he began asking and then pleading not to have to go to Mass. I guessed he must have drawn Judas.

On the day of the ceremony, I had virtually to drag him to the church. He tugged against me, wriggling continually all the way there; I just about managed to hold on to his sleeve as he tried to escape through his jacket. But then once we pushed on through into the vestibule, he kind of flopped down as a condemned man might on getting first sight of the unforgiving gallows. I never for a moment considered that Christopher might have become fixated on Judas's betrayal and hanging.

Thirty minutes after Christopher entered the vestry, the door creaked open and Father Monroe emerged (his nose preceding him), steadying a censer on a chain that belched plumes of smoke from its burning incense. His junior apostles, dressed in red or black cassocks and white smocks, hands clasped in prayer, trailed behind. All, including Christopher, were a perfect picture of rehearsed reverence.

There were grades of responsibility but the pinnacle of roles for an altar boy was the honour of ringing the tiny brass bell at the moment when the priest raised the host (the body of Christ) to celebrate the Eucharist. Christopher had been given that unnerving assignment. I sensed immediately the warmth of his palms, the tickling beads of sweat there and on the collar of his tunic. During the service he picked up the tiny brass bell much earlier than required and, overwhelmed by the weight of expectation, rang the bell in the wrong place. Mortified, he must have convinced himself there was no more ringing possible despite Father Monroe glaring at him to do so.

The service ground on. It must have been close to two hours before Father Monroe brought out the bucket of water for the washing of the feet. A fug of incense clouded over the steps leading to the altar where the stand-in apostles were arrayed in a single row kneeling in front of him. Apparently Father Monroe was bent on washing each individual toe. To help pass the time, I defaulted to my trick of imagining myself in command of a German U-boat, and giving the order 'Up periscope', I began to survey the congregation to determine who should be torpedoed. Half the enemy fleet had been destroyed when there was a collective stir over some commotion up front. I trained the periscope on the altar boys, now seated and bare feet washed; all except Christopher. My brother was still kneeling, bent over, and about to collapse. His head banged onto the ground and slid across a film of water on the floor.

I made my way out to the aisle, genuflected quickly to the statue of the cross and rushed to the front. Christopher was already regaining consciousness by the time I reached him. I noticed that the pool of water beside him was straw-coloured. I ushered Christopher to the vestry. And what he said there made perfect sense.

He'd simply wanted to go to the toilet but had become increasingly overwrought by the majesty and piety of the ceremony, and felt trapped, unable to move. When the priest finally reached him the delay and the sight of the bucket of water had been too much. Christopher had felt faint and could no longer control his bladder; he'd wet himself.

It might have been just as Christopher had said and nothing more sinister. It was to be our secret. But what if it had had more significance? What if the fainting at the Last Supper was his first sign of an affliction and had heralded his present condition? But then what would have been the value in bringing it all out into the open, and spoiling more than just the Mass but his whole childhood? Why deny him that? Unwittingly, perhaps, we had bought some more time, more years; years of not knowing that his life was spoilt and would never be perfect – far from it. Why alert the child to the onset of his epilepsy? He'd find out soon enough.

Epilepsy has been wedded to numerous epithets. At various stages in history words like 'degenerate', 'lunatic' and 'feeble-minded' have been hurled at people with epilepsy. Such derogatory descriptions were used without fear of censure throughout the centuries, and applied to prince or pauper. When Prince John, the son of George V, developed epilepsy, to shield him from the indignity of public scrutiny and to spare the blushes of the Royal Family he was secreted away to Sandringham, their private estate in Norfolk, and never mentioned again.[6]

Stung by the stigma, unsurprisingly, people with epilepsy did not disclose that they suffered from the condition. The nineteenth-century writer and illustrator, Edward Lear, kept a diary for all of his adult life. He was fastidious, rarely going a day without making an entry. The diaries are frank. He even made a note of his bowel movements. Yet there is one aspect of his life that was never recorded. Looking through the diaries you occasionally come across an entry which includes the letter 'X'. These were the days on which Edward Lear suffered epileptic seizures. With a closer reading, it's possible to work out that the epileptic days are also coded. Dotted throughout the diary a number sometimes appears beside the X – from 2 to 10, denoting the severity or longevity of the attack.

On Friday 19 August 1864, Lear wrote:

*Certainly — we fall. — And the dreary penalty comes on — weariness — sadness — apathy — foreboding — misery. **X**. at 2 P.M.*

But that seizure was at least an improvement on Wednesday of that week when he confided to his diary:

*(**X9**) ! ! Took medicine. Fretted.*

At times Lear appears to have had more than one fit in the day. The entry for Thursday 16 June 1864 begins:

*Awake at 4. **XX**. And back returns the Dark with no more hope of light!*

Throughout the diary he remains sanguine, soldiering on. But on days like Monday 20 June 1864 his pen was as exhausted as his spirit; he could only muster:

***XX** alas. —*

Occasionally Lear referred to his condition as 'the Demon' and, looking back over his life, he accepted phlegmatically that the Demon's constant presence from a young age 'would have prevented happiness under any sort of circumstances. It is a most merciful blessing that I have kept up as I have, and have not gone utterly to the bad mad sad.'

Edward Lear had had his first attack as a five-year-old child, but no one outside of his family knew of his condition or the shame that he felt about it. That shame was only offset by his sense of achievement and triumph in guarding his secret until his death.[7]

Lear's reticence would have been appreciated by the poet Emily Dickinson who had died two years earlier. Some condition had ailed her for much of her fifty-five years. The sparse medical notes do not lead to a definitive diagnosis, but a forensic analysis of her work suggests to biographers such as Lyndall Gordon that the 'It' at the centre of a number of Emily Dickinson's poems is epilepsy.[8] Further clues to the 'loaded gun' perpetually aimed at the poet and the internal volcanic explosions that threatened to disrupt her life are offered by lines such as 'I felt a cleaving in my mind—/ As if my Brain had split—'[9] that are seeded in the poems and course through her work, as obviously as 'Blood must follow vein', as my mother would say.

If the 'It' is both deficit and credit then that's because though the paroxysms constrained her, and led to her exile from society as a hermetic recluse in Amherst, they were also the source material of alchemical poetic experiments in the 'dying night' that Dickinson bequeathed to readers from her writer's cherrywood table in the room from which she rarely emerged.

But why the secrecy? For many years after her death (and before) the narrative told of Emily Dickinson to explain her seclusion was that she was a quaint and helpless young woman disappointed in love who sought refuge from that humiliation in her father's house. But the image from many of her poems, the repeated anxiety expressed over a loss of decorum and control, together with the pharmacological records of the prescriptions for her unnamed illness, present a compelling case that the seclusion was a consequence of the stigma Dickinson would have felt over her epilepsy; the shame of it and the fear of public humiliation propelled her from social gatherings up to the safety of her room. In nineteenth-century America's polite society, epilepsy was associated with syphilis, insanity and masturbation; in some American states not only was marriage ill advised, it was forbidden.

Emily Dickinson lived a domestic life but also an alternative, epileptic one. The duality she expresses in her writing is often shared by others who have the condition. Again and again she teases at that which cannot be written; she can only go so far in revealing how the reclusive suffering might ultimately lead to an exalted existence. In her visionary poetry, Dickinson comes close to showing but not telling of that alternative life located in epilepsy: 'And yet—Existence—some way back—/ Stopped—struck—my ticking—through.'[10]

Emily Dickinson's secret was kept by her family. No one broke rank; and there is so much secrecy that the truth is difficult or impossible to distil.

In her determination to 'tell it slant' in composing her poems, that is through metaphor, Dickinson's poems find echoes in the work of the contemporary writer Lauren Slater, whose book, *Lying: A Metaphorical Memoir* (2000), is an account of her epilepsy. But then again it isn't. For Slater is playing a sly game, having her cake and eating it, by suggesting early on in this meta-non-fiction writing that the truth, as well as the narrator, is unreliable. *Lying* may all be made up.[11]

In the book, Slater performs an impressive sleight of hand: she hides her epilepsy by revealing it, frankly – sort of. Any Jamaican, even if unfamiliar with postmodernist theory, would see straight away what she is doing. Jamaicans are schooled in the art of obfuscation. They call it 'playing fool to catch wise'. For hundreds of years it was a strategy that served their need to preserve an inner sense of self-worth and dignity when their daily lives offered constant humiliations and degradations during and beyond the days of slavery. Does Lauren Slater have epilepsy? What better revenge over your illness than to describe it and yet leave people wondering whether you were telling the truth.

I would later recognise this quality in Christopher, in his slippery and at times exasperating approach to his condition. For instance, he refused to wear the recommended metal bangle engraved with the word 'Epilepsy' which he dismissed as reductive, branding him an epileptic. If he had a seizure in the street, and was brought to a hospital's emergency unit, he would never own up the condition. The first time it happened, I was eventually summoned by the hospital. I arrived spitting feathers, angry and frustrated with him over what appeared to be a cavalier approach to his health and well-being. But on the walk back from the hospital Christopher described his seizure or the accident as a 'fall from grace' – and a very public shaming from which, in his own way, through playing fool to catch wise, he sought and found protection.

Epilepsy is spoken about much more freely today but has the stigma disappeared? My brother was not comforted by the roll call of famous historical figures that were thought to have had epilepsy. His attitude reminded me of the old Groucho Marx joke: 'I don't want to belong to a club that would have someone like me as a member.' But isolation is also corrosive – as has been shown by the story of Edward Lear and numerous public figures. In part, Lear's embarrassment about his condition was exacerbated by his embrace of his family's sense of collective disgrace. He was schooled in shame by an elder sister, Harriet, who acted as his tutor and believed the corrective approach to epilepsy lay in moral hygiene (desisting from masturbation), and that it might be eliminated altogether by self-control.

That notion of dishonour to self and family has diminished in Europe but it has proven more robust in places such as Egypt and China, where a self-loathing 'moral blame' pervades the households of families whose members are epileptic. There is no equivalent in the Chinese language to the English 'stigma'; a close approximation might be the phrase for 'loss of face'.

A measure of the shame attached to the condition can be gauged by the fact that up until four years ago, the official Chinese term for epilepsy was *deen gan tsing* ('crazy seizure disorder'). It was only in 2010, after almost a decade of lobbying in Beijing, that the name was amended to the neutral *no gan tsing* ('brain seizure disorder').

Because of the continued stigma associated with the disease, disclosure is still problematic for many epileptics. When it came to his employment prospects my brother identified with Yossarian from *Catch-22*: he found himself in a bit of a bind. The pattern was always the same. Christopher believed that if he fessed up about his epilepsy to a prospective employer in a job interview, he would never get the job. If he kept quiet about the epilepsy then he might be offered the post. But, having started the new job, eventually Christopher would have a seizure in the office. The first fit might be excused – if the employer was particularly sympathetic – but after the second seizure (perhaps a month later) he'd be taken to one side by his boss and asked not to return. I don't know how he stood it but he never complained. When I asked him about it, Christopher would just shrug and give his best Tony Soprano impersonation: 'What are you going to do? It is what it is.'

*

Opinion polls have revealed persistent prejudice towards people with epilepsy across time and place. Researchers in the USA in 1979 found that 18 per cent of respondents objected to welcoming an in-law into their family if he/she suffered from seizures. The figure was much higher in China where 87 per cent objected. But though the polls show cultural differences, there were also significant local and regional variations.

Had the USA survey been extended to include the population of New York's Little Italy, perhaps the results might not have been so encouraging. Judging from Martin Scorsese's *Mean Streets*, epilepsy still carried a heavy stigma in the 1970s. In the film, Charlie, the protagonist, played by Harvey Keitel, is having a clandestine relationship with a young woman called Theresa. Charlie goes to see his uncle, a Mafia boss, who has concerns about the company he is keeping – his 'half-crazy' friend whose mental state is not surprising, says the uncle because, 'His whole family has problems. His cousin, Theresa, the one who is sick in the head . . .'

'No,' says Charlie, 'she has epilepsy.'

'That's what I said,' answers the uncle. 'She is sick in the head.'

I was struck by the dialogue in that scene when watching the film soon after it came out. I would have a similar encounter with ignorance when discussing Christopher with my father thirty years later. Those prejudicial attitudes, so casually aired in *Mean Streets*, were not significantly different on the other side of the Atlantic, as was evident at about that time from the public furore over the revelation that the captain of England's cricket team was an epileptic.

Standing at six feet six inches, the batsman and captain of England, Tony Greig, presented an easy target for the Australian and West Indian fast bowlers, such as Jeff Thomson and Michael Holding. Tony Greig might have been a tower of strength, adopting a determined 'stand-to-attention' stance at the crease, but he had more difficulty than most getting out of the way of cricket balls coming at him like bullets at over 100mph. Batsmen could be battered and bruised after an encounter with the Australian and West Indian pacemen.

But Tony Greig had other reasons to fear an appointment with the cricket ball. He'd been diagnosed with epilepsy as a teenager: any kind of physical trauma, a knock on the head with a cricket ball for instance, might trigger a seizure. Yet Greig declined to wear a helmet – at least when first suggested, arguing that helmets would make cricket more dangerous by encouraging bowlers to bounce the batsmen. And anyway, he refused to be intimidated by fast bowlers or by epilepsy for that matter.

Outside of that bravura, Tony Greig had a sober and sensible approach to his condition. In his youth, he'd argued with his parents over their tendency to be over-protective:

'Maybe I was foolhardy, a stubborn martyr. But I was lucky. I came to no harm by carrying on just the way I had always done. I never had an attack while on a bike; I never passed out while swimming, and gradually my family realised that they would take half my life away if they insisted on chaining me with safety regulations.'[12]

Greig was tenacious, but he did fear the press and exposure. Even up to the 1970s there was a stigma attached to epilepsy that might exclude you from a number of professions – many more than the obvious ones, such as being a pilot. It was also inconceivable that the Lions of England would be led out onto the cricket pitch by an epileptic. Greig's epilepsy was a well-kept secret. If anything, among the conservative elements of the MCC, the prevailing view of Anthony William 'Tony' Greig, the South African-born cricketer, was that he was brash and aggressive – not quite English in his all-out professional determination to win.

More than detractors, though, the ranks of admirers swelled for the Cricketer of the Year, 1975. *Wisden*, the cricketers' almanac, was not alone in being impressed by the aura around Tony Greig. In its entry for the blond, blue-eyed captain of England, Wisden wrote admiringly, 'Here is the Nordic Superman in the flesh.' But like the singer and songwriter, Neil Young, the epileptic Tony Greig benefited from another kind of aura: the finely tuned sense of an oncoming seizure. At the advent of an attack, Greig would excuse himself and quickly find somewhere to retire discreetly; and prepare for what was coming. He also took the precaution of lying down in the pavilion and napping during the changeover from batting to fielding. It didn't always work.

Earlier in his career in 1970, making his debut for Eastern Province against Transvaal, Greig had an epileptic attack. His teammates huddled round and held him down until the fit abated; and the cricketing authorities managed to convince the press and the 8,000 spectators that he had merely suffered a bout of sunstroke.

After Greig moved to the UK, those broadcasters and journalists who knew about his epilepsy did not publicly comment on it; under the gentleman's code of the time it was a private matter. Even when the cricketer had another very public seizure at Heathrow airport a few years later the consensus held.

But when the captain of England transgressed in the eyes of a number of aficionados by throwing in his lot with the media mogul Kerry Packer's cash-rich, breakaway World Series – an ungentlemanly rival to the international cricketing board – the levers of social control seemed to come off. Henry Blofeld was one of the first commentators to break ranks when he alerted unsuspecting readers that 'there was an unwritten law . . . never to mention Greig's handicap'. In *The Packer Affair* Blofeld revealed the secret: 'Tony Greig is taking tablets for epilepsy, he's an epileptic and that may be one reason why he's made this ridiculous decision.' How else, suggested Blofeld, could you make sense of Greig's betrayal of the fine traditions of English cricket for the multicoloured kit-wearing, floodlit TV-recording of Kerry Packer's bat'n'ball circus?

Whilst others sought to distance themselves from this outbreak of journalistic indiscipline, they did so by airing the kind of prejudice which went some way to explain why Greig might originally have thought it wise to keep his own counsel about his condition. A reporter for *The Times* felt duty bound, for instance, to explain that 'Greig's impulsive behaviour and nervous mental energy' was a result of an illness which, though 'connected with the brain has emotional undertones'.[13]

Repeatedly in history, advances in the medical understanding of epilepsy have not been matched by a commensurate acceptance on the part of the public. In an omnibus survey carried out in the UK in 2001, informants were asked how and why epileptics were treated differently.[14] Many respondents thought it reasonable to exclude epileptics from employment 'because they might be injured or put other people in danger in the course of their work'. Liability at work was also voiced as a concern lest 'something went wrong and [the worker with epilepsy] wouldn't be able to do it properly'. The fear of being present in the event of someone having a seizure led to a determination that they would 'not socialise [with] or befriend them'. And it was understandable that 'normal' people were wary of epileptics because they were 'freaks'. A century after neurologists had sought to detach the condition from any stigma respondents still asserted their belief that epilepsy was 'associated with mental illness', and worried that such people were not 'in full control of themselves at all times'. And finally there was alarm that it was impossible 'to tell if a person in a seizure [was] drunk or on drugs' so that consequently 'people [were] afraid to get involved'.

Back in the 1970s, Tony Greig was initially furious about the way his epilepsy had been publicised; and that fury had not burnt out by the time he died in 2012. But in the decades between, Greig had turned his attention to disabusing the ignorant about the condition; speaking eloquently and openly, he would no more dodge a question on epilepsy than he would, standing at the crease, duck from a lethal cricket ball propelled by a fast bowler.

'So, how Christopher?'

'He's fine,' I answered.

'For true?'

'Yes, what are you getting at?'

'I hear him have some head trouble.'

The man speaking was my father. Bageye had been estranged from all of us (his wife and children) for thirty years. I had travelled to see him and broken the long silence. In his seeking to be debriefed, to be brought up to speed with the last three decades, the subject had turned to his youngest child.

'What? No.' I failed to disguise my irritation. 'Who told you that?'

'Is just what I hear.'

'No, he has epilepsy.'

'So, it true what them say?'

'What?'

'The head trouble him?' My father's voice was tremulous, apologetic and fearful. I had never known him to be afraid of anything.

'Him change up?' The old man wanted to know how Christopher had changed with the head trouble. 'How him look?'

My father was a Jamaican born in 1928. His perception of epilepsy would have been shaped and governed by superstition that ran like water through the island. People marked with head trouble were all the more scary because until they did something that revealed their condition it was impossible to tell them apart from anyone else.

Can You Smell Burning?

How does the story of epilepsy begin? For a large number of people with the condition the onset is a mystery. Nothing in their history has prepared them for the moment: it was not ordained. Epilepsy arrives into their lives without warning; as unexpected as it is unwelcome. But maybe there was foreshadowing that passed without recognition. Only later, retrospectively, might they piece together the clues. Perhaps it started with a smell. Consider the case of George Gershwin.

If the elegant frame of the celebrated American pianist and composer seemed always to be encased in a dinner jacket, then that's because this darling of the 1930s jazz scene – both of cognoscenti and of Manhattan's high-society bon viveurs who hoped for a sprinkling of his stardust – hardly ever refused an invitation to a party; neither did he have to be coaxed to sit down at the piano to enthral and delight the highball-swilling crowd. Populist and serious, in Anna Hamburger's words, Gershwin 'had the ego of genius and accepted the adulation that constantly surrounded him as effortlessly as his admirers accepted his ego'.[1]

In his starched shirt and spats, George Gershwin was a perfect emblem of the Jazz Age. Never far from a cocktail and with a fat cigar between his teeth, Gershwin mesmerised the guests at soirées with the brilliance of his songs and the virtuosity of his playing.

But his confidence was dinted in 1936 by the Broadway failure of the first outing of *Porgy and Bess*, prompting Gershwin to retreat to California. There he was dogged by a series of nervous complaints: the return of gastrointestinal problems that he called his 'composer's stomach'; and excruciating headaches that forced him to spend long periods lying down in darkened rooms.[2]

Performing with the Los Angeles Symphony the following year, George Gershwin suffered a near show-stopping moment that was far from scripted: in an uncharacteristic lapse of concentration, the maestro lost his place in the score. The momentary absence was covered up, but Gershwin was alarmed by it and confided to a friend that it had coincided with a nasty smell of burning rubber, which none of the orchestra, other than he, had detected. In another incident, which appeared to be related, Gershwin had had some kind of blackout and had nearly fallen off the stage. Reflecting on his poor state of health, George Gershwin now recalled other times he'd noticed a phantom smell, the unpleasant aroma of burning rubber.

He consulted physicians in California but they could find no organic problems, and he was diagnosed as suffering from hysteria. This would not have come as a surprise to those critics who'd previously labelled Gershwin a hypochondriac. An odour that no one else could smell might be just as disturbing as a voice that was inaudible to others but might also lead medics to reach for a psychological explanation. What neither his detractors nor the physicians picked up on, though, was the possibility that the phantom smell of burning rubber could be an 'aura', a type of olfactory hallucination commonly associated with temporal lobe epilepsy.

Aura is taken from the Greek for 'breeze'. In one of the early accounts of epilepsy, the ancient Roman physician and medical theorist, Galen, described the moment before a young sufferer's loss of consciousness: 'Just before he was no longer aware of himself . . . [there] was a movement upwards like a cold breeze.'[3]

In the second century AD, Galen (a celebrated physician initially to gladiators, and later to Emperor Marcus Aurelius) formalised the theory that man's well-being relied on the balance of four humours (fluids): blood, phlegm, yellow and black bile. Any excess or imbalance of one of the humours could lead to disease. Epilepsy was the consequence of black bile blocking the ventricles of the brain.

The 'cold breeze' of Galen's patient was the expression of a symptom physicians had noted but not yet named. In Galen's conception, there were three different categories of epilepsy: the first group related directly to the pathology of the brain; the second sympathetically related to the brain, originating in the cardia (heart); and finally the third group was related to the brain, but started in the peripheries. Epilepsy, then, could begin just as it did with the youth, as an 'aura' in the extremities that worked its way up through the body, spreading like a venomous poison. Such a belief underscored the practice of tying a ligature further up the limb from where the aura was first sensed in order to arrest the seizure.

For hundreds of years the Galenic model held sway. Lesser physicians were as likely to mount a challenge to Galen as today's junior house officer is to upbraid the senior consultant. If the theory of epilepsy evolved through arguments, then those quarrels were confined to the margins, as it were, of Galen's notes and medical histories, and centred on refining the details of his findings.

Today's neurologists would suggest that Galen's patient was articulating a sensorimotor aura. Technological advances in mapping the brain have enabled scientists to locate the specific parts of the brain that correspond to the sensory perceptions of auras; but the symptoms were first identified by Galen and those who came after him. In the first century AD, Aretaeus of Cappadocia catalogued premonitory indicators of epilepsy, such as hallucinations that preceded seizures. His list included 'fetid odours, luminous circles of diverse colour, noises from the ears, tremors and sensations in the hands or feet'.[4]

That ancient taxonomy is comparable to modern categories of auras; they include sensory (visual, auditory, olfactory, tactile), epigastric, psychic (déjà vu, jamais vu and flashbacks).

For the aura to be an aid to diagnosis it needs first to be recognised. The aura is the transmission but the signal is not always strong enough to be received. Perhaps the failure lies as much in its foreignness. Many people with minor absences from petit mal epilepsy can go for years without recognising that they have the condition. In his landmark study of over a thousand cases of suspected epilepsy, the nineteenth-century neurologist, William Gowers, recorded the case of a man with petit mal epilepsy getting dressed beside a bath. The man fell into the bath during a fit and got out of it again before fully regaining consciousness; he had no memory of the seizure, and only gathered that something was amiss because his suit was drenched.[5]

The failure to pick up on the signals also applies to friends and relatives. Quite often, of course, there is nothing obvious to detect. My mother paid forensic attention to our health during our childhood. Illness was an enemy to be guarded against. More than any other person that I knew, she was governed by her senses. Throughout the 1970s she was especially tuned to a sense of foreboding and the physical effect it had on her. The skin just below her right eye would twitch. It was a sign. 'My bad eye a-dance,' she would warn of some imminent misfortune. Her voice would be apologetic, low and grave. At the time, I considered it just one of her strange West Indian sayings and a feature of her temperament. Medical school gave me another way of assessing the phrase.

The dancing eye was just a tic, a twitching of the facial nerve below the eye and indicative of the need for a bit more calcium in her diet. But she was not convinced. Her bad eye continued to dance, as it did one morning in June 1983. My fifteen-year-old brother, Christopher, was in the bathroom and had failed to come out. He'd been inside for half an hour and hadn't answered our raps on the door or enquiries about how much longer he'd take. For the last ten minutes we'd grown increasingly anxious. As more seconds passed, my mother began pacing outside the bathroom. 'My bad eye a-dance,' she warned. 'I see trouble in this house tonight.'

It wasn't that easy to break down the door. Even when the lock was sprung, Christopher's fallen, unconscious body blocked the entrance. Our curiosity over the cause of the strange fainting paled, though, beside the relief that he soon regained consciousness and that we had discovered him fully clothed with his dignity intact.

There was no history of epilepsy in our family. It was just bad luck, but for some inexplicable reason our mother blamed herself – as if his medical destiny was within her grasp and not in the lap of the gods. After the first attack, the only certainty was that the seizures would come again. As Gowers spelt out a hundred years earlier, 'the occurrence of one fit facilitates the occurrence of others . . . [and is] to some extent the cause of other fits . . . Without that cause the disease might have remained latent for ever.' The epilepsy genie had escaped the bottle.

But the aura is at least an early warning of the seizure that's on its way; it gives those who receive the warning a chance to prepare themselves for the inevitable. The classification of auras has changed very little since the nineteenth century. Olfactory and auditory auras rank amongst the most prominent; and their descriptions over the decades since are often uncannily familiar. The revolting smell of burning rubber or rubbish figures in numerous descriptions of olfactory auras. Gowers observed that a number of his patients compared the unpleasant sensation to sulphur and to burning putrid meat. Medical literature abounds with case studies of seizures apparently summoned by the peals of phantom church bells. Auras are mostly repugnant and distressing, but occasionally there are accounts of welcomed hallucinations. In 1894 the *British Medical Journal* carried a report of a hospitalised patient made miserable, he said, by the ward's musical box that played constantly throughout the night. But in the last week of his life, the nurses recalled how he would drowsily 'lie on his back with a pleased smile on his face, keeping time with one hand to imaginary music'.[6]

Nineteenth-century neurologists traced the roots of auras to electrical discharges in the corresponding sensory centres of the brain; hallucinations involving bad smells, for example, were consequences of excitation in the olfactory centre of the cortex. Auras marked the beginning of certain kinds of seizure. But what prompted them? The next generation of neurologists would investigate further not just the sensory perception of seizures but whether sensory stimuli could trigger epileptic attacks. In doing so, they were entering territory previously only charted by hearsay and old wives' tales; such as the claims made in antiquity for the magical properties of jet, when the mineraloid was routinely thrust under the noses of slaves on the auction block by their prospective owners to determine whether they might be susceptible to epilepsy.

By the 1950s neurologists were investigating myriad accounts of epilepsy allegedly brought on by sensory stimuli. One patient, whose list of triggers ranged from air-raid sirens to the cry of a particular news vendor, included 'notes from trumpet and saxophone' in his final tally. It should not have come as a surprise to his physicians. Epileptic attacks brought on by music were first chronicled by Macdonald Critchley twenty years earlier in a paper focusing on music and the brain; outlining the case for what became known as musicogenic epilepsy.

Critchley's sample included patients who voluntarily demonstrated how their fits might be induced through music.[7] As a record of Tchaikovsky's *Valse des Fleurs* played, one patient recalled, 'My insides seemed to turn right over. My arms and legs went cold and numb from below upwards.' She could not resist the oncoming fit. Another found that a particular musical note would spark a fit; and yet another that simply thinking of a tune might set off a seizure. Critchley conceded the difficulty of disentangling a psychological component from the attacks when he included the case of an ambitious violin student who, on hearing that she had failed a critical exam upon which her career depended, fell unconscious; subsequently she suffered convulsions whenever she heard the violin played.

Neurology, perhaps more than other medical disciplines, is built on storytelling and the art of extrapolating general rules or truisms from particular case histories, whilst remaining alert, of course, to the possibility that the individual tale may be aberrant and not reflective of the whole. Neurologists guard against the seductive powers of the remarkable, yet at the same time are drawn to fantastic tales of the unexpected, as Odysseus's crew might have been drawn to the sirens had he not taken the precaution of plugging their ears with wax.

The remarkable case of the woman who captured the attention of the highly regarded neurologist, Robert Efron, is equally astonishing for the enthusiasm with which it was met by the profession.[8] Before detailing the case, Efron prefaced his paper with a defence of his predecessor Gowers, whose work on stimuli to arrest seizures had largely been neither embraced nor critiqued by his peers. Gowers was one of the pioneers of English neurology and the reticence of his contemporaries owes as much to their regard for him as to their nervousness and embarrassment of his exploration of a subject that was formerly the preserve of the folklorists and the superstitious.

In 1881 Gowers claimed, 'Attacks which begin by a general or bilateral aura, or by the epigastric sensation now and then may be stopped by some muscular exertion, as by walking quickly about the room, or by a strong sensory impression, such as the application of ammonia to the nostrils, and sometimes by the inhalation of nitrite of amyl.'

Efron, it seemed, had been pipped to the post by seventy years. But rather than being deflated by his demotion from leading man to supporting cast, Robert Efron was buoyed by the notion of his famous predecessor's work validating the importance he placed on his own primary research. Efron had also been inspired by the 'unusually articulate and analytic description . . . [offered] by [his] introspective patient', a forty-one-year-old professional singer; and he set down her case report in meticulous detail.

Mrs T.B. in describing her many seizures stated:

They are all like cars coming off the assembly line. I can't tell one from the next. I can be perfectly well in every way when suddenly I feel snatched away. I seem to feel as if I'm in two places at once but in neither place at all. I can read, write and talk and can even sing my lyrics. I know exactly what is going on but I somehow don't seem to be in my own skin. It is like being outside a room and looking in through a keyhole . . . After this has gone on for some time, I seem to get to what I call my halfway point. I feel like a piece of clay, inert. I don't try any more to prevent the convulsion. I push all the furniture away so I don't hurt myself when it happens. I suddenly get a smell like an explosion or a crash. Then I hear a voice off to the right calling my name, Thelma,

Thelma, almost as if it wants me to turn to it. No matter how hard I try I have never been able to keep from turning. Finally there is a big jerk and my head swings to the right, my right arm flies up. That's it. I'm out.

Efron imagined that Mrs T.B.'s description of the stages preceding an epileptic attack corresponded to the neural pathway along which the wave of excitation spread over the surface of her temporal lobe, culminating in the fit. And he postulated that he could interrupt that pathway by introducing a powerful sensory stimulus at the critical time (the patient's halfway point) before the olfactory hallucination was fully realised.

He proposed that Mrs T.B. inhale ethyl n-butyrate, but she found the smell too similar to the actual hallucinatory sensation and suggested instead that she be given a drug whose odour was its polar opposite. The patient was told to sniff a vial of hydrous sulphide (a mix of hydrochloric acid and ferrous sulphide). Remarkably, on the majority of occasions (the test was repeated seven times) the intervention worked; the seizures were aborted.

Efron also confirmed that the cessation was the result of the smell and not some innate pharmacological property of hydrous sulphide. He gave her a new drug with the same smell but made from entirely different chemical components. The outcome was equally compelling.

In her description of 'being outside a room and looking in through a keyhole', Mrs T.B. had also revealed a startling aspect of some kinds of epilepsy that had long intrigued neurologists and had led men such as John Hughlings Jackson to propose a hierarchy of auras. Sensory hallucinations, such as smell and sound, were crude auras; whilst the sense of being present and withdrawn at the same time constituted an intellectual aura – Jackson preferred the term 'dreamy state'. In this mental state of altered perception, patients had double consciousness: their consciousness was impaired, and yet at the same time they had the unsettling sensation of perceiving events which seemed to have occurred previously (reminiscence, déjà vu); or they experienced peculiar, unfamiliar feelings (jamais vu).

It was this dreamy state that accounted for Fyodor Dostoevsky's strange confession about his epilepsy that he made to a friend in 1836: 'For several moments I would experience such joy as would be inconceivable in ordinary life.'[9]

Déjà vu, though, is common in ordinary life – in people who have no pathological or neurological imbalance. It is unlikely to be considered a presenting symptom of epilepsy. Whether epileptic or not, we attach psychological or spiritual significance to déjà vu; and hardly see such altered mental states as cause for consultation with a physician.

In the 1930s neurosurgeons attempted to locate the site of the electrical discharge responsible for the dreamy state, and for déjà vu sensations. The change in neural function of epileptic patients with these reminiscences was identified when surgeons passed probes into the brain and found that a past experience, which had occurred regularly as part of the patient's seizure pattern, was reproduced by electrical stimulation of the cortex of the temporal lobe.

'I can tell when it's coming sometimes because I'll start to feel like I'm under water sort of and my hearing goes a bit.' The clouded consciousness of the dreamy state was a regular characteristic of the seizures endured by Brody, a seventeen-year-old student with ambitions to study music at university. She was my first interviewee and I was struck immediately, when she met me at the door, by her shy luminosity. Brody had recently been featured in a national newspaper, and her proud mother seemed as enamoured of her intelligence as the paper had been; but there was a protective instinct, too. The delicacy between mother and daughter suggested that Brody had had a recent seizure, but it might just have been transference on my part. Her mother hovered at the edge of the interview, just managing to stop herself from finishing her daughter's sentences. Brody was gracious with her. I was thankful to see such tenderness.[10]

Brody had volunteered for a video telemetry trial at London's King's College Hospital which involved her wearing electrodes that monitored her EEG and videoed her non-stop over a seventy-two-hour period to ascertain whether epileptic seizures might explain why she woke up after sleep to discover herself with black eyes and bruises. The video showed her in the throes of fits banging on the bedpost, falling out of bed, then returning to bed and snuggling back under the duvet without her sleep being disturbed. Brody had previously been diagnosed with both generalised and petit mal epilepsy. During waking hours loud noises, such as the bang of a burst balloon, might trigger an attack. But she also had auras – at which time she would reach for music as a balm.

'Music is a way that I can get away from the epilepsy,' she explained. 'When I have a tremor, brought on by the epilepsy, music allows me to escape that. It's almost as if when I'm playing it's not really there, and it's a way that I can cope and manage my epilepsy. So when I don't feel well or say I feel shaky, I will go into my room – and I will play the piano, messing about with different chords that I like, and my tremor will stop, my shaky feeling that I'd have previously will go.'

Aside from her own music therapy, the video telemetry was helping her doctors to fine-tune the amount and dosage of drugs she needed to take.

*

In the decades that followed the strange case of George Gershwin, neurologists were more likely to make the connection between mental absences and auras, whether olfactory (burning rubber) or the epigastric sensations which might have accounted for Gershwin's 'composer's stomach', rather than simply the butterfly nerves some musicians suffer from ahead of a performance.

Soon after his discharge from hospital with 'hysteria', George Gershwin sank into a coma; his deteriorating condition led to an urgent search for a neurosurgeon to perform an emergency brain operation on a suspected fulminating tumour and save his life. The news captivated people around the world. At one stage it involved the White House and a chain of surgeons who were either too far away or too nervous of their failing skills to act.

The unfolding drama of Gershwin's last hours undoubtedly influenced the film-makers Michael Powell and Emeric Pressburger a decade later when they embarked on *A Matter of Life and Death*.

Michael Powell, in filming *A Matter of Life and Death (AMOLAD)*, in which a Second World War pilot survives a crash but develops an undiagnosed neurological condition, was aware of the stigma of epilepsy and was always a little coy about using the word. 'I don't think I ever stated what was wrong with the young flyer (David Niven) after he's crashed in the bomber. A previous injury had caused adhesions on the brain . . . probably I didn't state it too much because many people had bangs and bumps during the war and you didn't want people to get too worried.'[II]

There was something wrong with Peter D. Carter, the character played by David Niven. He wasn't cracked or anything like that. No, God forbid, the English squadron leader was a spiffing fellow, a phlegmatic and heroic pilot who at the fag end of the Second World War jumped from his burning Lancaster bomber (without the luxury of a parachute) and miraculously survived the thousand-foot fall into the sea – enough to give a chap a few bumps. Carter suffered occasional headaches in the left temporal lobe region of his brain thereafter. That wasn't his main complaint though. After all, by rights he ought to have been dead. What disturbed him more and was distinctly odd was the smell of fried onions. He couldn't find where the smell was coming from. It was a sensation without a source; and one that Carter was beginning to realise signalled the onset of the hallucinations he'd started to have following the parachute-less jump.

Ever since its release in 1946, *AMOLAD* has both unsettled and intrigued viewers. Watching it as a child two decades later, I felt but never quite understood its beguiling effect on me. Back then, lacking a concept of hallucinations, I nevertheless grasped that something peculiar was happening to Peter Carter – in his head perhaps; events were taking place in space but not in time. The on-screen action stopped. But though the film was frozen, Peter Carter was still able to walk about, trying and failing to rouse his now statue-like friends. But he was not alone. In a twinkle, a heavenly messenger appeared: a foppish eighteenth-century French aristocrat, Conductor 71, tasked with collecting and conducting the newly departed from earth to heaven. Conductor 71 came to claim our hero. But since Peter Carter's miraculous fall from the sky, the pilot had tumbled into love and was reluctant to leave. To prove he wasn't cracked, Carter, his lover and the local neurologist devised a scheme: he was given a tiny bell to alert them whenever the heavenly messenger appeared.

Early on in the film, Carter drowses in a chair in the doctor's study, with the bell by his side. There comes a moment, so subtle that viewers might not realise it, when his nose wrinkles like the goodly witch in the TV show *Bewitched*. He must be smelling something. Fried onions? Of course! A gentle wind courses across

41

the screen; and a dirge sounds on piano, chords of foreboding. Peter Carter rings the bell but it is silent. What does it all mean?

Like many first-time viewers I suspected something but knew not what. Now it is clear that the film-makers were sowing the seeds of clues about the neurological condition of Peter Carter. The smell of fried onions, the wind, the music; all denoted the aura which precedes the hallucinations of complex partial seizures; and herald the epileptic incidents visited upon the traumatised pilot. Powell and Pressburger were precocious film-makers. *A Matter of Life and Death* was, for many viewers, simply a light-hearted and witty romance, but it was also a landmark pioneering film in the depiction of the disturbing neurological depletions of epilepsy. The sequences of freeze-framing, of the sculpting of time, are a subtle approximation for the hallucinations marking Peter's auras.[12]

In anticipation, Dostoevsky dreaded the aura's arrival; yet in retrospect he valued the ecstatic quality of some of them. The experience was unique. But the majority of epileptics do not experience anything close to Dostoevsky's ecstasy; and for them the value of the aura, whether olfactory, auditory or dreamy state, is not clear.

Pioneering neurologists such as Hughlings Jackson conceded that the dreamy state was probably no more than 'slightly raised activity of healthy nervous arrangements consequent on "loss of control" '. He cautioned that these dreams or fleeting transplantations to another world did not present in epilepsy without other symptoms, but he worried that they could still be overlooked. Dreamy states and accompanying symptoms such as chewing and spitting or the vertiginous feeling of objects moving closer and further from you might seem trivial but it could be that the 'patient has the serious disease epilepsy in a rudimentary form until a severe fit comes to tell him so'.[13]

But for many whose epilepsy is established, the aura, heralding a seizure, is nothing more than that. It's too close to the event to act as a warning; or to give time for the epileptic to prepare. It is simply portentous and cruel. It allows the epileptic to receive the warning but not to transmit the news to anybody else in time.

In the first phase of my brother's epileptic life, he never gave off any signals of an approaching seizure, apart from on one occasion when he rose before breakfast and asked, 'Can you smell burning?' But there was no bread in the toaster or bacon in the pan. He stood up in his slippers and immediately crashed into a fit.

For a while a pattern became discernible in the onset of Christopher's seizures. The 'danger time' was always the mornings, soon after he woke up. In the early days after his diagnosis, there was always a critical moment between 5 a.m. and 6 a.m., after which you were in the clear. If he had not had a fit by 7 a.m. he was unlikely to have one. I tried to intuit the likelihood of a coming fit in his face – or in a subtle change in his mood.

Our mum had her own sensors. Her bad eye would dance and she would be compelled to sound the warning as a deep dread overtook her body. And even after 7 a.m. she would not concede that the danger had passed for now because, 'The day long.'

I would keep close to him, discreetly so, and be ready to catch him or more likely break his fall. Christopher never spoke of any further auras, but over the years of scrutinising him I seemed to have developed an understanding with Christopher, a kind of sympathetic aura in lieu of his own, or at least I was never surprised when a fit did occur.

My brother and I also shared a delight in *A Matter of Life and Death*, especially after his diagnosis. In the film, as previously mentioned, the undiagnosed epileptic pilot is desperate to share his peculiar condition with his fiancée and doctor; and for them to be alerted and primed for his next epileptic attack. Asked to

43

describe what happens before the seizures, Peter Carter recalls that as well as the smell of fried onions, he kept on hearing the overture to *A Midsummer Night's Dream*. Both auditory and olfactory auras mark Peter's neurological episodes, but the signal is frustratingly unique to him: the others do not hear or smell it.[14]

But are there other predictors of epilepsy? The ancient Greeks thought so. They believed the cycle of epileptic attacks followed the expansion of the moon; attacks were more likely to occur in the build-up to a full moon. And there were also seasonal variations. The incidence of epileptic fits spiked during spring and also on rainy days. A rainy spring must have been a double whammy.

Epileptics can tell you that there is usually some general pattern to their fits; perhaps they've worked out that the seizures occur, like Christopher's, in the early hours of the morning. Increasingly, the kind of video telemetry undertaken by Brody is being exploited to chart the unique pattern of a person's heightened electrical activity and to gain a better understanding of the relationship between sleep and epilepsy.

Over the years patients have even tried to trigger their attacks so that the seizures occur at a more convenient – or at least less embarrassing – time, offering temporary, prophylactic respite. In 1959 the neurologists Falconer and James described a patient who 'rubbing the right side of his face with the back of his right hand, [evoked] a sensation that would continue spontaneously in a rhythmic and pulsating fashion and end in a seizure ...The patient made practical use of his knowledge, and would retire to a convenient place and provoke a seizure in order to prevent such an occurrence in awkward situations.'[15]

The anxiety of not knowing specifically when a fit will occur can be debilitating. It might introduce an element of caution into people's lives, especially when travelling; and might even deter some epileptics from leaving the relative safety of their homes.

But at the very least, the epileptic aura is a metaphor for fore-boding. What if, instead of releasing waves of anxiety and trepidation, the aura was converted into a measurable early-warning system? That was the jumping-off point for researchers at the University of Melbourne, who have gone a step further than the neurologists at King's College Hospital in developing a device that can be implanted onto the surface of the brain to monitor long-term electrical activity. Fifteen volunteers signed up for the trial. Electrical signals, giving continuous EEG recordings, are transmitted from the device and relayed wirelessly to a hand-held receiving monitor. This monitor will give a flashing reading on the screen of differing colours and vibrate when there's an alert, providing a kind of digital aura for the person with epilepsy. A flashing red warning light, for example, signals that a seizure is imminent.

This will not stop epileptics from toppling over, but perhaps they would be able to make themselves comfortable first. The implant in one volunteer had recorded just over a hundred seizures whereas the volunteer himself had recalled only eleven of them. Technology often attempts to solve a problem by mirroring a function of nature. The researchers liken what they are attempting to earthquake early-warning systems: 'You can't stop them,' says the researcher Mark Cook, 'but if you knew when one was going to happen, you could prepare.' In eleven of the volunteers the device successfully predicted these imminent 'red-light' seizures (likely to arise within four minutes) two-thirds of the time.[16] But will the trigger from such a device to the monitor be any faster than the organic aura of burnt toast or the signal that elicits premonitory tremors in the hands?

Others are more inclined to trust their own memories of these fleeting warnings: 'Before you slip into that other world,' says the singer Neil Young, 'you start to feel all weird and echoey.'[17] In that phoney period before the fit, the queer feeling reminded Young that he needed to do something about it. He had 'about forty-five seconds' before the window of opportunity closed.

Unlike Peter Carter, George Gershwin did not survive the last-ditch operation to remove a suspected tumour. Eventually the chief neurosurgeon at the University of California operated on Gershwin at 5 a.m. on 11 July 1937 but to no avail. Within a few hours of the operation the composer was dead.

The confusion over Gershwin's medical condition highlights the aura's potential importance not just as an early warning of a seizure but as a possible key to making a correct diagnosis in the first place.[18] It may not have affected the prognosis for Gershwin as his signs and symptoms of seizures were themselves brought on by the fulminating tumour. But as many doctors have subsequently testified, recognising the sensorimotor auras earlier on could have bought some time for Gershwin and his physicians. In the build-up to 1937 a battery of medics failed to heed the warnings, and clarity was eclipsed by organised confusion.

The Visitor

How do we picture epilepsy, especially if we have never seen someone having a fit? What imagery do we draw on to locate and understand it? When epilepsy is mediated through film and television the portrayal is often graphic, and no more subtle than the way it is rendered in religious tomes such as the Bible. What hope is there for anything other than a clumsy understanding of epilepsy when the representations are so crude?

Was Christopher cursed with head trouble or blessed with an opportunity for God to show his mercy? Our grandmother, we were soon to learn, took the latter view. If you were inclined to put the mystical before the medical then you would have found comfort in her company. I recall the North London house – a kind of rum shop fused with a nunnery – where she lived with several of her adult children, with all of its contradictions. Welcoming wafts of cinnamon (from all of the baking that went on) were often pushed out after the evening meal by the sweet fug of ganja; the King James Bible competed on the dining table with partially filled-out coupons for Littlewoods Pools and the *Racing Times*; and unguarded, ribald tales of big-voiced men burst through the background hum of religious fervour which though understated could at times be suffocating.

Usually, Grannie Reid sat to one side in silent communion with herself. She had come to that house in Kenton in the 1970s from Jamaica (via Luton) with four or five children. The numbers varied because although there was a steady core, one or two were itinerant; they came and went either because of the vagaries of their merchant seamen's lives or because they'd fallen in or out of favour with the clan. All were strong and impressive characters but it was obvious that power resided with the little old lady in the corner whose body and prayerful lips twitched with mischief day and night. Grannie Reid was a seer. She had a gift that was rarely spoken of but was acknowledged by all. She could 'read' people. She heard and saw things that no one else could sense. She had a third ear and, more importantly, a third eye.

Some remark must have been made to our grandmother about Christopher's condition because one day, soon after his diagnosis, he was summoned to lunch. Fearful of what she intended, I offered to accompany Christopher. We turned up late because he had an epileptic turn that morning.

Grannie Reid was sitting in her usual spot with a large bible open on her lap, flanked by a couple of elderly friends, but paying no attention to them. Her eyesight was good yet she traced a finger over the sentences, as though the words were Braille that she could feel through her fingertips. Enlightenment might come through reading the Good Book, but a gloom of permanent dusk pervaded that house. Some kind of social pathology was always at large throughout its rooms. Matters of health were endlessly mulled over: an innocent birthmark of someone out of favour was rumoured to be a leftover trace of syphilis; tales abounded of treacherous English doctors who if they got their hands on you, 'you finish' because they liked nothing better than to 'experiment on black people'; herbal 'bush' tea was brewed up and administered as a 'good wash-out' of the system for every ailment; and other old-time remedies from back home were advanced as a corrective to the NHS's medical negligence.

I felt we'd entered a trap; that, in agreeing to come and see her, we'd taken a wrong turn. On the doorstep, Christopher and I made a whispered pact that we'd leave on the first suggestion of any blessing, before the ritualistic holding of hands or the humming of sad hymns.

Grannie Reid closed the bible as we came through the door, and although she looked up in our direction, she seemed to see beyond us. She called for hush, flapped her arms and hands in a further gesture for quiet from our aunts and uncles, and the myriad Caribbean folk for whom the house was a hub. She pointed to my brother, and the rest of the room followed her gaze. A warm and knowing smile played on her lips.

'You see! Can't you see? You see the light above his head?' she whispered. 'You see the light? Jesus is here.'

Writing now, I recognise that for decades I told that as the climax of a story about me. I softened it and gave it a quirky but benign twist – as an example of a child's inability to live up to a grandparent's expectations; but Christopher claimed the story too, and rightly so. Perhaps like many siblings we so often tried on each other's anecdotes that we sometimes lost sight of their provenance.

I can see how Grannie Reid's vision – 'You see the light above his head? Jesus is here' – was in keeping with her belief in a miracle to rescue Christopher from his 'affliction'. It was inevitable that she would frame his epilepsy in such a way. Her bible was a guide and handbook for life. The text written in a font which suggested antiquity, the extra-thin pages rimmed with gold and the heightened colour of the illustrations (imitations of Renaissance paintings) deepened her reverence.

But we had no understanding of the history of art; and though we suspected the images were an approximation of something else from another time, we had no conception that they were the work of an artist. It might well have been Raphael's paintings reproduced in the bible, but up to that point I had not knowingly seen his work, and neither had Grannie Reid, I imagine. And yet in trying to make sense of Christopher's epilepsy she had drawn on a biblical tale whose imagery had been rendered with much pathos and so movingly by Raphael: the transfiguration – now made manifest in Kenton.

The Transfiguration – a dual painting of the risen, recently crucified Jesus Christ in the top half, and apostles and a crowd focused on a stricken boy possessed by devils in the bottom half – was the final work of the Renaissance master, Raphael. It is one of the most significant portrayals of epilepsy in the history of art. Commissioned as an altarpiece in 1517, *The Transfiguration* was hailed by the early art historian, Giorgio Vasari, as Raphael's 'most beautiful and most divine work' – a description given added poignancy when, following the Herculean task and nearing its completion, the thirty-seven-year-old Raphael succumbed to a fever in 1520 and died.[1]

The Transfiguration was a work designed to inspire devotion – seeing and believing through contemplation. The religious imagery in iconic altarpieces underscored the grand ambition of Renaissance artists such as Raphael to conjure a visionary experience for the viewer and to provide a portal to another, spiritual world. But the real power of *The Transfiguration* lies in the tension of its unusual composition.

In the upper zone of the huge thirteen-foot-high oil painting, Christ in billowing white robes floats above Mount Tabor. Miraculously, he has risen again after his crucifixion; alongside Moses and Elijah he is transformed and exalted, emitting a light so radiant you'd need to shield your eyes. It is a scene of triumph.

Below, on earth, in the lower half of the painting, there is darkness and desolation. A distraught father supporting his son in the grip of the 'sacred disease' pleads for help from the apostles; and they, unable to cure the boy, beseech Christ to intervene.

The boy's head is thrown back; his eyes have rolled upwards so that little more than the whites remain. He is unbalanced and arched backwards as he falls. His limbs are flexed and contorted. Both arms are flailing. But though dramatic, the painting is imbued with pathos. Raphael's *Transfiguration* is sympathetic to the plight of the boy who, in the biblical tale, is presumed to be suffering from demonic possession, a view of epilepsy that still prevailed in the sixteenth century. The symbolism of the trans-figured Christ is contrasted with the naturalism of the pitiful scene of anguish around the sickness of the fallen/falling youth. Over centuries critics have struggled to interpret the painting. Goethe, writing on the unity of the painting, suggested that 'below are those who are suffering and need help: above is the active power that gives succour'.[2] And for Friedrich Nietzsche the harrowing suffering of, and around, the boy was a depiction of 'primal pain'.[3]

In recent years historians and physicians have argued over whether the boy is in the midst of a seizure or rather recovering and cured. In 1995 a *New York Times* headline trumpeted 'Cardiologist Answers a Raphael Question'. Dr Gordon Bendersky was credited with decoding the mystery that had perplexed scholars for five centuries.[4] Citing the boy's open mouth as evidence, Bendersky contended that the painting depicted God's clemency and healing: 'It was traditional to show a demon or a small cloud emanating from the open mouth of an epileptic at the end of the spasm. This was supposed to be the casting out of the unclean spirit. Thus, the boy's open mouth depicts the devil escaping rather than the boy emitting a cry during a seizure.'

But no matter the stage of the seizure or Raphael's sympathetic portrayal, the artist does not question the notion of demonic possession. The transfiguration stops short of transformation.

Throughout much of human history, the depiction of people with epilepsy did not change; they were unquestionably possessed. Sometimes, as in *The Transfiguration*, Jesus was invoked to drive out the demon. It is not difficult to understand that mindset. Even today, people undergoing grand mal seizures appear to have been taken over; as if their bodies have acted as vessels for some foreign occupation or alien invasion. Electricity snakes through them; their body snaps like a bullwhip. And then they're back to normal. Or are they?

They seem alien; they might look like us but their bodies have been invaded and then snatched from them. They are people like us; but then they aren't, not really. For centuries people with epilepsy have suffered from this problem of perception – their own and others.

For all the times I studied Christopher's face as a child I could not foresee his future. There were lots of opportunities. Our mother, reminding us that it was 'she one lef' for bring up all us pickney', encouraged the idea that 'one finger can't crack lice' by farming out the responsibility of putting the youngest to bed. During those years of his infancy I lay down beside Christopher, cheek to cheek, at six o'clock and waited for him to drop off. Unfortunately, he'd quickly worked out my treacherous habit of slipping away when he slipped off into sleep. Thereafter, he took to holding on to my earlobe as he slept. There was nothing for it but to accept that this was the way it would be and to endure. I'd look for the subtle changes in his cheeks, the eyeballs rolling underneath the lids, the relaxing of his throat, the shallowness of his breathing. Only after thirty minutes, sometimes more, would I be able to ease my earlobe from his grip, to stand and try to determine which floorboards would betray me as I crept away. But even then I'd turn to watch over him; I loved the carefree way he slept. I spied on him, delighted in his face.

At the beginning of his adventure with epilepsy, the condition had no bearing on Christopher's expression but over time, following each fit, some vestige of it remained in his eyes – a quality of distraction, of retreat and internal migration. It was a look I'd only ever previously seen on very old people or the recently bereaved. Occasionally, he'd sense me scrutinising him and without turning to face me he'd say, 'I'm going to start charging, you know. A pound a glimpse. A fiver a long hard stare.'

I wanted to discover what it was that marked him with epilepsy; and whether there was some transference in my being able to see the epilepsy in him because I already knew that it existed – the way people would say retrospectively on meeting a stranger who turned out to be epileptic that they 'had a feeling'; that they knew something wasn't quite right. 'Ah, now you say so and so has epilepsy, so that explains it.' Fyodor Dostoevsky alludes to that feeling in *The Idiot* when early on he offers the reader a description of his protagonist, Prince Myshkin: 'His eyes were large, blue, and piercing, and there was something gentle but heavy in their look, something of that strange expression which makes people realise at the first glance that they are dealing with an epileptic.'[5]

Dostoevsky had only to look in the mirror to test the truth of that observation. Years of fits had left an imprint on his face, but perhaps only those who looked closely might recognise it. Psychiatry teaches us that we can develop selective perception when it comes to areas of life that impinge directly on us. Exposure to his own epilepsy had made Dostoevsky more perceptive to its effect on the visages of others. Some medics, with years of experience in treating epilepsy, make the same claim. But to me they're as reassuring as the doctors I met in my first years at the London Hospital who, alerting their colleagues to a difficult child who'd exhausted the medics' descriptive powers, might scribble in the notes the abbreviation 'FLK' which they and all the physicians understood as 'Funny Looking Kid' though no one knew what it actually meant.

In describing Myshkin's eyes, Dostoevsky seems to be referring to the trace of previous fits that might eventually disappear if there were no subsequent attacks. Dostoevsky was not so lucky; fits shadowed him for much of his adult life. When Dostoevsky's bride-to-be first met him she was struck by his enigmatic expression and the dissimilarity between his eyes: 'One was obviously brown and the pupil in the other was so dilated you couldn't see the iris at all.' Anna Grigoryevna, though, was not given to fanciful thoughts. She did not see Dostoevsky's eyes as windows to his epilepsy. One eye had been damaged when, following a seizure, he fell on a sharp object. And in her reminiscences his wife offered the prosaic explanation that the permanently dilated eye was a consequence of the atropine drops he'd been prescribed.[6]

The commonly held belief is that epilepsy subtracts from a person, physically and emotionally, that it's a downgrade, but Dostoevsky challenged this notion in several novels. He asked, what if at some level it's an upgrade? Prince Myshkin might appear to be simple but he is actually extraordinary, and the impact of epilepsy on his character and how others perceive him because of it lies at the heart of *The Idiot*.

Dostoevsky began writing the novel under enormous stress. In the autumn of 1867 when he sketched out the character of Myshkin, he was on the run. He had fled Russia to Europe with his new bride to escape the demands of relatives, swindlers, loan sharks and a host of creditors who were snapping at his heels. Throughout his adult life, he'd taken risks, gambled and reeled from one financial disaster to the next. Even outside Russia he continued to gamble at the roulette table and to lose heavily. Writing *The Idiot* was one last roll of the dice. It was his 'get-out-of-jail' book: the newly remarried forty-five-year-old was depending on it to turn his fortunes around.

But his seizures knew no boundaries. They followed him abroad. 'As soon as I arrived in Geneva,' he confided to a friend, 'my fits began. And what fits! Every ten days a fit and it took me ten days to recover from it.' Between the seizures somehow he managed to write, and after half a dozen false starts, the character of Prince Myshkin, in whom Dostoevsky saw himself, began to emerge. But the writing took a heavy toll: 'The finale [of the first part],' he later recalled, 'I wrote by inspiration, and it cost me two epileptic fits, one after another.'[7]

Prince Myshkin is the idiot in question in the novel; he is perceived as such by most, if not all, of the major characters as an innocent, a village idiot, albeit a titled one. Dostoevsky sees him quite differently. To the author he is saintly, a Christlike figure, a Russian holy fool.

But it was not the transfigured Christ of Raphael from whom he took inspiration. Rather it was Hans Holbein's portrayal of the brutalised, putrefying corpse of Christ taken down from the cross and encased in a claustrophobic coffin which so disturbed the writer that it could, as one character in the novel suggests, have caused a Christian to lose his faith.

Anna recalled how, in Basel, her husband had been transfixed by Holbein's painting of the dead Christ. He stood rooted in front of it for fifteen or twenty minutes, held captive by its realism and horror. And he later mused that surely Christ would have wavered in his sacrifice had he been shown, as the painting so graphically depicted, the appalling end in store for him. Dostoevsky stared so intensely at the dead Christ that Anna feared her husband was on the verge of another seizure.

The Dead Christ rekindled in Dostoevsky an old idea that had possessed him for a number of years: to write about a 'completely beautiful human being'. Myshkin is self-effacing, with, seemingly, an underdeveloped ego. His epilepsy sets him apart. Sent away as a child to a sanatorium in Switzerland, he returns, still poorly, but is now the mysterious beneficiary of an inheritance. His privilege and good fortune, though, are no protection from the seizures that erupt at moments of unbearable tension throughout the book. *The Idiot* was set contemporaneously in the latter half of the nineteenth century and it's clear that Dostoevsky meant the fragility of Myshkin's epileptic body to mirror the underlying fissures of Russian society that threatened seismic change to the existing order and the primacy of the aristocracy. But if his epilepsy is a liability it is also his salvation. Myshkin's personality is informed by his condition; he remains a marginal man, on the borders of the corrupted aristocratic world but not of that world.

Violence, death and near-death haunt the book; and if in Myshkin's grand mal seizures we see the rehearsal for death, we also see that the lucidity of the pre-epileptic aura experienced by some such as Dostoevsky and his protagonist is akin to the clarity of vision of the condemned man on the eve of execution who has lived in the shadow of the gallows.

Dostoevsky humanised people with epilepsy at a time when his contemporaries were more likely to demonise them. Even an author as sophisticated as Dickens could not resist the temptation to assign negative and criminal characteristics to sufferers of seizures. In *Oliver Twist* the reader could be forgiven for concluding that the hideous Monks's affliction is an obvious manifestation of his evil. Whilst Nancy primes the reader with a simple unprejudiced description of Monks's epileptic appearance, 'His lips are often discoloured and disfigured with the marks of teeth, for he has desperate fits', at the book's finale, Mr Brownlow rounds on Monks with a damning analysis linking his criminal personality to the 'hideous disease which has made your face an index even to your mind',[8] namely epilepsy. But was Monks also a prisoner of his biological inheritance?

Hysterical notions of a criminal class swept through panicked Western societies in the nineteenth century. But it was also an age of cataloguing and classification, of exciting scientific developments which held out the prospect of answers. Following its bloody unification Italy was especially receptive to some of these ideas. From the defeated south, murderous brigands roamed the countryside, sending waves of terror north and throughout the country. The ruling class was perplexed and rejected the 'apologist' view that social inequalities might explain the violent fallout from the war. Far more attractive was the view expressed by the neuro-psychiatrist Cesare Lombroso, that 'the degenerate is a product of diseased ancestral elements which ceased to evolve progressively . . . so that pathological individuals manifest rudimentary physical and mental attributes of primitive man'. Lombroso appeared to break new ground with his compelling hypothesis of an atavistic criminal class, a subspecies of humans, throwbacks whose physical appearance bore closer resemblance to primitive man.[9]

By Lombroso's scientific reckoning (he'd studied hundreds of skulls), born criminals could be identified through their physiognomy, the bumps and contours of the cranium, the size of ears or protrusion of the jaw. But thrilling though they were, Lombroso's ideas (written up in *Criminal Man*) did not constitute an all-encompassing theory. A number of anomalies threatened to undermine his theory. No quantity of cranial bumps could explain the diversity of pathological behaviour among criminals. Perhaps, he surmised, a hidden agent arrested the development of particular organs such as the brain. Lombroso delved deeper and settled on epilepsy as the contributory factor – the root of criminality lay in the combination of atavism and epilepsy. All atavistic (born) criminals were epileptic, though not everyone with epilepsy was a criminal.

Cesare Lombroso's hypothesis was widely adopted by pioneers of modern criminology (he was esteemed as its founder).[10] 'Lombroso's Theory of Crime', a 1912 paper published a few years after his death, broke off from its fulminating praise of the master to propose that his teaching suggested that in order to combat degeneracy and crime it was essential to deal with epilepsy, and that if society agreed on the need to segregate the insane, then the same must surely apply to 'all pronounced epileptics'.

Today it seems bewildering that such titanic confidence could emerge from research that largely relied on anecdotal case studies. Initially, in the matter of epilepsy and atavistic criminality, Lombroso leaned heavily on the case of Salvatore Misdea, a young soldier with epilepsy, who in 1884 had run amok in his military barracks, killing a number of his colleagues. Called as a medical expert, Lombroso judged that 'Misdea was bearing in the face, in the skull and in his habits, the features of the born criminal.' And as he pondered what troubled him about the case, the sudden unbidden thought arose that the soldier's great criminality 'was a form of equivalence of epilepsy'. Subsequently Lombroso wrote, 'I began to rummage among epileptic skeletons and skulls and I found the same proportions in the median occipital dimple and in the facial asymmetry that [others had] found in the skeletons of born criminals.'[11]

Five years later, Lombroso's expertise was also called upon to cast light on the relevance of epilepsy in the case of the anarchist Luigi Luccheni, the assassin of the Empress of Austria. Lombroso judged that the 'very brachycephalic' Luccheni, with his 'half-closed eyes, roundish ears, heavy eyebrows, voluminous cheek bones, jaw prognatic [and] low forehead', had a number of characteristics 'of degeneration common to epileptics and insane criminals'. And further, Lombroso concluded gravely that the assassin's denial of hysterical epilepsy was 'already a beginning of a proof of disease'.[12]

Later, and for decades up to the 1930s, photographs of sufferers of epilepsy with facial asymmetry would be analysed anthropometrically and offered as supporting evidence in criminal court cases.

In the catalogue of anthropological photographs that supported the thesis linking epilepsy with criminality and primitive man, again and again people with epilepsy are framed as starkly as the subjects of police mugshots. Even without a placard or identifying number plate, the images are harsh and unforgiving. Such photos may have disappeared from the public domain but the prejudices they underpin have remained. Often it has fallen to artists with epilepsy to challenge these domain assumptions.

In casting a former supermodel, Agyness Deyn, in the leading role for the 2014 film *Electricity*, the film-makers attempted to confound our expectations about the face of epilepsy. The young female protagonist, Lily, reels through the film on amber alert, half-expecting another fit at any time. *Electricity* visualises and captures the swirling spectral lights of Lily's hallucinations, her interrupted memories and the fractured quality of her life. Lily's attitude towards her fits is phlegmatic: 'Thrash get up get on with it.' Again and again she crashes face down onto the floor, and subsequently, the mirror can only offer a clue to the bruised and bloody consequences of what has befallen her; the real horror is reflected in the pitiful gaze of those who witness those harrowing seizures.[13]

By the very nature of epilepsy the seizure and its aftermath are stages that barely register on the consciousness of someone who has suffered a fit. They are spared the indignity. But video telemetry trials such as that conducted by King's College in London afford people with epilepsy the opportunity to see just what happens to them when they are having a fit.

'In the majority of seizures the patient has no recollection – everybody else knows apart from him or her,' says the neurologist Professor Franz Brunnhuber. 'Some are intrigued and want to know exactly what they're doing or hopefully not doing during a seizure. They may then profit from knowing how others may respond to them.' But Professor Brunnhuber concedes that 'other patients are too scared or are not ready to see them'.[14]

Brody fell into this camp. 'I haven't looked at the recording, no,' she said when asked. But she wasn't alarmed at the prospect, she wanted me to know: 'It's just it seems that if I was to look at it I wouldn't know what to make of it.' Brody spoke lightly. The simple fact was that she'd 'rather not know about what happens during them'.[15] She would not be drawn when I pressed a little further. Brody was disinclined to engage in thoughts that might unsettle her; and I caught a glimpse of how she must have been as a younger child, dreaming up a personal code to transcend difficulties that adults might try to insist on talking about. Children cope in this way: why talk about a future danger when you could circumvent it by avoiding the cracks when walking on a pavement or holding your breath until the car you were in reached the end of the tunnel?

Professor Brunnhuber believed that some patients, at the other end of the spectrum from Brody, felt liberated by the knowledge gained from watching themselves when playing back the video telemetry. 'They themselves may have bizarre or unjustified feelings about what they are doing,' he said. 'For instance, there are complex partial seizures where someone may just be lip smacking and have no recollection for a period of one to two minutes, and some patients are quite relieved to note that actually not much can be seen. It can start the process of further understanding one's disease.'

The recordings have a ghostly CCTV quality and some patients describe how they feel distanced from the subject of the footage (conceiving the person on the screen as someone else) and even begin to feel tender towards that apparent stranger in their vulnerable state. But it was understandable that a teenager such as Brody, notwithstanding her maturity, might be unable to do that and be disturbed by the results.

And Brody is right. For a person with epilepsy reviewing an attack it is difficult to know what to make of the strange wooden choreography of a seizure; to fathom what happens to your delicate thoughts as your consciousness is barged out of the way by a force that comes from within and explodes outwards. The chance to investigate what had been an abstraction, before the advent of video telemetry, was not inviting to Brody; far better to be left in ignorance, without the peculiar ocular proof of instances when your life and body spiralled out of your control.

'Control' is the key word in epilepsy. Even though epilepsy is very common, most people will never witness a person having a seizure. Film, the most popular art form in the twentieth century, is likely to be the medium through which many of us gain an understanding of the condition. But the consultant neuropsychologist Sallie Baxendale believes that if film is an index of cultural awareness then the signs are not good. The last seventy-five years have witnessed a progressive trend towards more explicit depictions of epilepsy, says Baxendale, in which 'erroneous and dangerous stereotypes are perpetuated'. This is especially evident in male characters with idiopathic epilepsy in films such as *Deceiver*, *The Terminal Man* and *To What Red Hell*, who are portrayed as 'deranged and dangerous' and out of control.[16]

In a paper published in 2007, Toba Kerson, a professor of social work and social research, set out to explore the extent to which, in over a hundred films in which epilepsy features, 'audiences delight in and are titillated by others' loss of control'. The films, in a number of different languages, include quirky shorts such as *Le Déshabillage Impossible* and blockbusters such as *The Exorcist*. They range from the subtle to graphic depictions, and from sympathetic to exploitative portrayals. Though it's impossible to draw conclusions about differing cultural stances towards epilepsy as revealed by a few film-makers of a variety of nationalities, the films do chart and perhaps mirror society's shifting attitude towards the condition over the years.

The pioneering French film-maker Georges Méliès is credited with the first filmic depiction of epilepsy in *Le Déshabillage Impossible* (*Going to Bed Under Difficulties*), 1900. Acting in that film, Méliès fails to take off his clothes and go to bed because every time he removes an outer garment miraculously another appears; jacket, shirt and trousers are instantly replaced, again and again with increasing speed, matching Méliès's fury and frustration until he collapses into a seizure. George Méliès's intentions are purely comic; the magician/film-maker is more interested in the virtuosity of the technology and in substitution tricks than in an exploration of multiple identities and personalities that some critics and scholars divine in the two-minute film. Nonetheless there is much to be gleaned about attitudes and prejudices from the unintentional and from tangential approaches to epilepsy in films.

There's a fleeting moment in Terrence Malick's *The Tree of Life* when a central character cradles and shields her infant son from the sight of a neighbour having a seizure on the lawn. It's a marginal scene: there is no comment on what is happening – just some men gathered around the man fitting on the ground and the mother with her hand covering the infant's eyes. But that episode captures succinctly the parameters of 1950s USA and the disquiet over any departure from the mythic safety of suburban

life. Unsightly epilepsy did not fit into the idyll. The scene is
framed so that the seizure takes place at the margins of the screen
and seems to occur almost out of sight. You might catch it out of
the corner of your eye but blink and you'd miss it.

Few films focus on the effect of epilepsy on an individual's life
and character. Anton Corbijn's *Control* is an exception. No feature
on the rock musician Ian Curtis who killed himself at the age of
twenty-three in 1980 could skirt round his epilepsy. *Control* tackles
it head on. The title is a play on one of Joy Division's best-known
songs, 'She's Lost Control'. The founding member, Bernard
Sumner, recalls that the title came from an incident involving a
girl (a job seeker) at a rehabilitation centre for people with physical and mental disabilities where Curtis worked: 'She had epilepsy
and lost more and more time through it, and then one day she
just didn't come in any more. [Curtis] assumed she'd found a job,
but found out later that she'd had a fit and died.'[17]

For many, a diagnosis of epilepsy can be devastating. Coming to
terms with it is not unlike the stages some go through when told they
have a terminal illness. In her book, *On Death and Dying*, the
psychiatrist Elizabeth Kübler-Ross posited a theory which she
called 'the five stages of grief': anger, denial, bargaining, depression
and acceptance. The singer Ian Curtis seems to have navigated a
number of these stages in his short but consequential life.
Ultimately, he travelled along a road between rejecting and
embracing his disability.

In 1980, Ian Curtis took a kitchen line, wrapped it round his
neck and hanged himself. In the film this grave step follows on
from the grand mal seizure that he suffered the night before. Even
though his story is necessarily truncated in *Control* the film makes
a strong case for the correlation between his epilepsy and his
decision to kill himself. It is as bleak as the black-and-white images
of Macclesfield's urban landscape, the deprived northern English

town where Curtis was born. The film is dour and uncomplaining (like its subject): it doesn't want to make a fuss; and yet it is vital, too, especially delighting in those moments of performance when the taciturn Curtis is transformed into a forceful dynamo of distilled poetic expression. He *was* a rock star, after all. His was a melancholic but luminous voice that had enthralled a generation of music lovers. And here again was a personification of a tragic life cut short – an anthem for doomed youth. Ian Curtis's suicide sowed the seeds for a cultish nostalgia amongst fans for the sound of their own youth (doomed or not) and a mourning for what might have been.

Joy Division passed me by. In the late 1970s and 1980s, my ears were more finely tuned to reggae; but the extraordinary appeal that Curtis and his band held over my peers was strikingly apparent, a fascination that has continued with another generation, exposed to the enigma of Ian Curtis through documentaries, feature films and myriad profiles in music magazines.

A large part of the fascination is tied up with the feeling that Ian Curtis's creativity was underscored by the mysteries of his epilepsy – a condition that was allied to the otherworldliness of his on-stage persona, and that gave a clue to the revelatory power of his music.

The first time I watched Ian Curtis, as thin as a Giacometti statue, fronting Joy Division on the band's John Peel recording session in 1979, it wasn't long before I was tempted to look away. It felt voyeuristic. He seemed peculiarly both fired up and spectral. The febrile, greyish skin that would have been clammy to touch was at odds with his youth. At the recording he was twenty-three but seemed younger; a gangly adolescent who had yet, perhaps, to come to terms with a recent growth spurt. Curtis was one remove from the rest of the band. Of course, it's hardly unusual for a lead singer to distance himself – he is after all the focus of attention – but Curtis was not aligned with the other members: his planet did not share their orbit.

All of this was intuited from the TV archive; from the immediate suggestion of his deep immersion in the song and its mood; before this gave way to the sickening thought that Curtis was only a few clicks from losing control of his body, reeling like a punch-drunk boxer. Thank God for the mic stand, I thought. The singer was not just grasping the microphone; he was being propped up by the stand. When he ripped the microphone from its holder and abandoned the stand I feared the worst. His eyes glazed over; when the delicate lids closed there was only one place those eyes could have gone: to the back of his head.

On stage Ian Curtis was continually on the move; he was known for the strange convulsive spasms that branded and burned through his performance; at times they mirrored a man in the throes of an epileptic seizure determined not to fall down. But Ian Curtis did fall down. Epilepsy felled him; it had sent him crashing off the stage in the midst of a Joy Division gig the year before and on numerous occasions thereafter. He was discomfited by his epilepsy; and yet he exposed his fragility for audiences to see and to be equally discomfited. This was not the anarchic yet choreographed pogo-jumping thrashings of punk; this was a public airing of a very private grief. Curtis's performance was an expression of his epilepsy and his art. Through it he revealed an extraordinary ability to transmit a profoundly felt emotion. According to his wife Deborah, his dancing had become a 'distressing parody of his off-stage seizures. His arms would flail around, winding an invisible bobbin, and the wooden jerking of his legs was an accurate impression of the involuntary movements he would make.'[18]

Ian Curtis's seizures were an acute manifestation of a chronic but treatable condition. Before treatment, though, comes prevention. Why did Curtis do nothing to limit the effects of his epilepsy?

That which should have been avoided was embraced. Sleep deprivation, from touring the country in the back of vans, and free-flowing
alcohol, were accomplices which brought forth seizures in the
singer again and again.

And neither did the range of medical options appeal to him.
For many years there had been no effective treatment for epilepsy.
The first generation of anti-epileptic drugs, offering partial relief
to some patients, were only developed in the late 1930s. For much
of his life Ian Curtis refused any prescribed pharmacological intervention. Though his recreational drug regime was extensive, it did
not include Epilim (sodium valproate) or any other anti-epileptic.
On the surface he appeared reckless, but Curtis was petrified by
the probability of drugs altering the delicate balance of his mind.
He did not want anything, neither drugs nor his condition, to
control him.

When he did relent and take medicine, band members recall,
the results were alarming. He suffered violent mood swings.
Working on an album in 1980, he was gripped by a claustrophobic
feeling of being pulled down into a vortex; of drowning in words
that were writing themselves. Now, not only was his body channelling his epilepsy, but so too were the songs.

Curtis was not nihilistic. But the potential to lose control, to
surrender to fate and the furies, was alluring. Who doesn't, on
some level, at some stage, yearn to let go, to roll around in the
gutter, freed from the constraints of keeping up the charade?
Which epileptic wouldn't dream of being given a pass, of escaping
from his or her fractured life? My brother certainly did. His relationship with the drugs were like that of an addict, inversely so.
He was on again; off again; on; off. When we nagged him about
his propensity to stop the medication, he'd promise to get back
on it straight away. But his default position was one of anger: he
was vexed about the need to have to continually take the drugs.

Ian Curtis was angry about love; yet he wrote searing, heart-rending love songs. He was angry about the seizures and the toll that they took on his mind and his body; yet he laid bare its ravages in performance. He was angered by the brutality of epilepsy, by its indifference and randomness. He couldn't be in control. It was out of his hands. And yet his death, when it came through suicide, was evidence of a man struggling to take charge of his life and wrest control from epilepsy. In the notes that Curtis kept with one of his lyrics at this time, he wrote, 'Even the flames from the fire seem to beckon me, drawing me to some great past life buried somewhere deep in my subconscious, if only I could find the key . . . if only . . . if only. Ever since my illness, my condition, I've been trying to find some logical way of passing my time, of justifying a means to an end."[19]

Control is a fine film but in its unremitting and gloomy depiction of epilepsy it does a disservice to people with the condition. There is, however, a scene early on in the film where the seriousness looks as though it is about to be leavened by humour. Ian Curtis, in his day job working for the council, interviews a woman who brings along her daughter to the meeting. Inexplicably, the child wears a padded helmet (the kind worn by boxers in training). In the midst of the interview she falls down and bangs her head. The child has epilepsy; and the helmet is a precaution. Perhaps comedy would not have been in keeping with the tone of Joy Division's music or Curtis's life but the reverence is overdone. The scene foreshadows Curtis's lack of protection and preparedness. When he collapses in performance, Curtis is carried by his band members from the stage like the wounded in battle or Christ taken down from the cross.

There is a tendency (and I am especially guilty of it) to bestow a kind of nobility on people with epilepsy. Dostoevsky asks the reader to consider that in Prince Myshkin at least this might just be justified. Myshkin has an attractive, ethereal quality, and if you looked closely I'm sure you could see signs of him in Ian Curtis. I certainly saw Myshkin as a kindred spirit of my brother. But this is simply transference, surely; the kind exhibited by liberal white Americans in 1960s Hollywood movies who assigned nobility to the quietly suffering but dignified 'Negroes'; the kind that assuages you of guilt for the pity that you really feel for these exemplary candidates for compassion.

Pity was a response rejected by my brother. As his epilepsy progressed, Christopher adopted a fixed attitude towards it. He preferred to make a joke of his condition, and encouraged me to do the same. After that particularly volcanic seizure on the morning of our trip to Kenton, I'd sat with him for a very long time. That period immediately following a fit and before he regained consciousness was always a strange, phoney, liminal state.

The transformation, when the seizure finally left him, even though you knew it would come, was always remarkable. It was a joy to behold; and I was as relieved and awed as any parent who has kept a night-time vigil beside his sickly, febrile child and is present when miraculously the fever breaks.

Eventually, Christopher's eyes opened. He seemed confused as to what had happened.

'You had a visitor,' I said.

'Yeah?'

'He's gone now.'

'What did he say? Any message?'

'He said he'd come again.'

I am Me No More

J is delicate and petite, perhaps a few inches taller than five feet. Her size is important: more than once she alludes to it as one reason why strangers have treated her with such kindness following a fit – the others being that she is middle class and well-heeled. When we speak she holds my gaze in a manner that suggests the quiet confidence of an actor used to attention. She is not an actor, but an artist with an extraordinary and shocking tale to recount.

A decade ago J was violently assaulted in North London. The national newspapers reported how, when cycling near her home, she was attacked by motorcycle muggers, knocked off her bike and left with a serious head injury. She was rushed to hospital, in need of an emergency operation for an epidural haematoma, and in a critical condition. The prognosis was poor. She fell into a coma. Over the next few days and weeks, J's parents were summoned on more than one occasion as the doctors, believing J would not survive, felt duty-bound to offer her parents a chance to pay their last respects. But J endured the surgery (a craniotomy) and recovered; and after months of treatment and incremental improvement she was discharged from hospital. Everyone hailed her miraculous recovery. But there was one final twist to the story: months later, as a delayed consequence of the assault and the traumatic brain injury, J developed epilepsy.

I asked her what she recalled of the attack and she said simply, 'They took my identity. They stole my identity.' I assumed she was speaking about her loss of memory following the mugging or the psychological effect of the trauma which had left her with a new unwanted identity as an epileptic. But in fact J had simply meant that the muggers also took her bank cards and identification papers.[1]

She smiled graciously at my mistake. It appeared at first that she was not much given to introspection. She was happier to talk about concrete details – and even pulled back her hairline (without me asking) at one stage to reveal the metal plate just beneath the surface of her skin that was required following surgery to keep her skull together.

J hadn't meant 'They stole my identity' metaphorically but it would have made sense if she had. There is an element of confusion that accompanies some forms of epilepsy. The temporary aphasia of the man who was 'Just awake', or the amnesia of the patient whom Gowers reported had fallen into the bath during a seizure and climbed out again without any recollection as to why his suit was wet, is not uncommon. There's a sliding scale of interrupted consciousness following some seizures; and the automatic subconscious action (automatism) can range from lip smacking to more complex mechanical movements akin to sleepwalking.

J's petit mal seizures could be especially troublesome if she was in transit. 'Sometimes I'll get on a Tube and end up somewhere I really didn't mean to be.' She spoke precisely, casting herself as a dotty old aunt. Her self-deprecating ('silly old me') manner reminded me of my brother. And although she spoke in the first person the evenness of her voice distanced her from what was being said: she sounded as if she was describing somebody else.

She suffered from both grand mal and petit mal seizures. But although the grand mals were dramatic and potentially dangerous,

J found the smaller absence seizures to be more problematic because she was unable to explain to anyone what was happening: 'I will feel terrible but unable to ask for help because I can't communicate. It's frightening because sometimes it's a lead-up to a grand mal seizure so I feel like at any point I could fall over, but I can't act on it. I appear quite normal – I will stand up. I might look a bit frustrated but I just . . . Communication just breaks down. It's a bit like being underwater. It's like some part of the world has changed. So it might seem that my movements seem really slow and what I'm saying is not what I think I'm saying.'

In the immediate aftermath of a seizure state, when consciousness is occluded, people with epilepsy can make few decisions for themselves. It's a terrifying predicament, as Prince Myshkin notes early on in *The Idiot*: 'I always lapsed into a total stupor, lost my memory completely, and though my mind worked, the logical flow of thought was as if broken. I couldn't put more than two or three ideas together coherently.'[2]

To understand what is going on during a seizure when consciousness is interrupted we first have to distil how consciousness arises. Despite huge advances in neurophysiological research scientists are still struggling to interpret the meaning, for instance, of the neuro-imaging signal changes that are registered during an epileptic discharge.

Whether the seizures are generalised or partial, it is clear that impaired consciousness results from a disruption of the complex neural networks that allow for consciousness. Fundamentally, in general seizures there is decreased cortical activity and increased activity in other regions of the brain, such as the upper brain stem. The resulting altered state of the brain has two components: modification in the level of consciousness; and alterations in the content of consciousness (subjective experience). Following on from a fit, people with epilepsy often find that these latter,

71

peculiar changes to the qualitative characteristics of consciousness are impossible to describe.

Unsurprisingly, artists have been drawn to exploit the drama that is inherent in such moments. Raymond Chandler turned expediently to epilepsy in a plot device for his novel *The Big Sleep*, which centres on Carmen, a young woman who, in the aftermath of a seizure, shoots a man but conveniently can't subsequently recall anything about the incident. Chandler hints at the concept of automatism, the idea that a person might commit an unconscious act (as noted earlier in some incidences of epilepsy), and is therefore not responsible for the consequences of that act. In criminal law automatism has been advanced by lawyers as a mitigating factor in their clients' defence. When Marlowe, the cynical private detective, sets eyes on Carmen he is not convinced: 'She seemed to be unconscious but she didn't have the pose of unconsciousness. She looked as if, in her mind, she was doing something very important and making a fine job of it.' But *The Big Sleep* is a thriller and not a high-minded work of literature teasing out the nuances of motive and mental states. Chandler is determined that Carmen's neurological condition should not distract readers from the fact that the girl with the smoking gun is also a nymphomaniac.[3]

Nonetheless, no matter how crass its depiction, *The Big Sleep* shows one of the truisms of epilepsy, in the way that at least temporarily after a seizure the sufferer has no option but to rely on the judgement of others. The results are hopefully benign but not always so. Sometimes the unexpected consequences are malign, and even catastrophic.

There was a period before Christopher had been given a definitive diagnosis when our mother still held out hope for divine intervention. 'I fast and pray, fast and pray,' she would proclaim whenever

I broached the subject. 'What else can I do? Can a mother's tender care cease towards the child she bears?' One day when I had my own children, she said, I would understand. Miraculously, the prayers seemed to pay off – a year or more went by without another incident. Even so, the prayers did not stop but the focus shifted. Instead of calling upon God to stop the fainting, she implored Him to prevent Christopher from passing his driving test.

Before he was even old enough to drive, Christopher had become obsessed with buying, renovating and selling second-hand cars. He learnt how to change brake pads, to tune an engine and to wire in a cassette player. By his eighteenth birthday he'd upgraded from the first £100 junk cars to a shiny Alfa Romeo that he had no intention of selling; and then God failed my mother. Christopher passed his test.

That same day my mother reported that she had gotten a 'little vex' when Christopher prepared for his maiden voyage. She insisted that he should not go out in the car alone. She grew further enraged when he refused to answer her, even after she'd snatched his newly purchased driver's gloves from him. It wasn't like him to be 'so ignorant' she said, but he had simply stared blankly at her. Frustrated, my mother left the (one-sided) argument but a while later she returned to find Christopher by the front door (now wearing his driver's jacket), fiddling endlessly and repetitively with the lock. Oddly, he did not leave. A partial seizure had interrupted the maiden voyage, it seemed.

It was a couple of days before I could get to Luton to answer my mother's questions about Christopher's bizarre behaviour. She stiffened when I used the word 'epilepsy'. 'I don't want to hear that name, not today.' And though I was beginning to doubt that it could be anything else I too refrained from mentioning the name again.

In the months to come we would substitute the word 'turn' for seizure or fit. If I telephoned for a progress report, she'd whisper into the mouthpiece, 'I think it happen again,' or, 'It seem so that t'ing still trouble him.'

Her uncertainty stemmed from a lack of familiarity with the character of the turns; they varied. Before some pattern was established it was difficult to work out when or even *if* he had had a seizure. The generalised ones seemed obvious to me. I suspected that partial complex seizures (like on the day of the maiden voyage) were also thrown into the mix. But the absences from these seizures were difficult to distinguish from what was becoming a characteristic of Christopher – a conscious decision to shut down, to become unresponsive.

That was especially the case when it came to the car. Christopher continued to pursue his favourite hobby in the teeth of opposition. We all counselled against it, but he was adamant.

A week later there was another neurological lapse. In a repeat of the one-sided argument (with me now replacing my mother) Christopher moved automatically from dull-eyed absence to determined (almost seemingly predetermined) action. I don't doubt now that it was some form of automatism. My mother paced around the kitchen wailing that her bad eye was dancing and that she foresaw trouble ahead. She implored me to do something, to say something. But words had no effect: they bounced off Christopher as I trailed behind him out of the house and onto the street. Finally we reached the point where we were standing alongside the Alfa Romeo. Christopher opened the car door and got in.

The magnitude of what was happening, and the speed of it all, was beyond me. It brought on a sudden sickening fairground ride of emotion – a shearing-away of certainty. My mother stood helpless in the arch of the front door in great distress, willing me not to abandon her baby son to his fate. I dreaded that look. I'd seen it in the imploring eyes of parents investing all hope in the consultant on the eve of an operation on their child. And it reminded me of a friend who was terrified of flying. The friend once described how her fear had drained away when she saw two famous musicians board the plane after her. It was impossible to conceive that that great iron bird would fall out of the sky with Kylie Minogue and Nick Cave on board. My mother was of similar temperament. No matter how great her anxiety she was inclined to believe that nothing bad would happen to Christopher so long as *I* was in his company. She would never have asked me directly to get into that potential death trap with him, but she expected it of me. I could not refuse.

In a fury, I jumped in and slammed the car door behind me, cursing my stupidity. But finally I reasoned with myself that Christopher had never (to my knowledge) had two fits back to back in one day; and in any case once I was sitting next to him in the passenger seat, he'd come to his senses: though he might risk his own life, he surely wouldn't risk endangering mine. How strangely the order of things was reversed. It was as if I was underwater now and he, carrying on with his normal activity, couldn't hear me.

Christopher thrust the key into the ignition.

'Don't. Don't do this,' I said.

Even if he publicly denied the diagnosis of epilepsy, Christopher must have suspected it. And for good reason people with epilepsy are forbidden from driving. Loss of consciousness is not compatible with driving. People have been killed in the past; and negligent perpetrators jailed. In Britain you need to have proved that you have been free of fits for two years before your licence is handed back.

'Don't be a fucking idiot!' I said.

He started the engine and we took off. I continued to shout at him. My arguments grew increasingly desperate, like a jilted lover making one last attempt to dissuade his soon-to-be-ex from leaving him. My mother's foreboding rang in my ears: 'I see trouble in this house. Trouble. Trouble, O Lord.' Three or four minutes onto the M1 motorway I noticed that Christopher's eyes had started to twitch, and then they were blank. As if on ice, the car slid across the motorway from the outside lane to the inner one, and finally sank into a ditch. Miraculously, no other car was involved, and neither of us was hurt. A few vehicles pulled up behind us. Three or four men emerged and helped me to push the Alfa Romeo back onto the hard shoulder. I drove us home. My mother was still at the front door. I brushed angrily past her into the kitchen and threw the car keys into the bin.

The next day Christopher had no memory of the incident. Jokingly, he offered me a lift to the station. 'Has anyone seen my car keys?' he asked. Nobody answered. He patted the pockets in his trousers and jacket. He began searching his room and then every room in the house. His humour soured. He complained that somebody must have stolen the keys. No one answered. Eventually Christopher confronted me and I confessed what I had done, and that the bin men had come and emptied the rubbish that morning. He was apoplectic.

'If I can't drive, what can I do? It's me. Driving is me!'

'Not any more,' I said. 'It's all over.'

'Not any more?'

'You're not driving any more,' I said drily.

'I am. I bloody well am.'

'No, Christopher, you're not. Not any more.'

'You know what you've just said?'

'What?' I barked. 'What have I said?'

'You don't even know what you said. You said, "you're not any more". You're saying I am me no more.'

On the few occasions when Christopher would consent to a frank conversation about his condition, I would often invoke the names of great figures who, in spite of their epilepsy, had led rich and rewarding lives – Van Gogh, Julius Caesar and a host of others. The response was always the same. 'Van Gogh and Caesar!' Christopher would laugh sarcastically. 'And how did it work out for them?'

Julius Caesar suffered at least four recorded episodes of epileptic seizures. They all came in the last two years of his life when he was already in his fifties. The late onset was atypical. Epilepsy was more commonly believed to be a disease of childhood and puberty because it appeared to cease after marriage. This led some to advance the logic that sexual intercourse could be a cure and should be encouraged early on, even if, as the Greek physician Aretaeus complained, it 'did violence to the nature of children by unseasonable coition'.

For centuries, physicians have wrangled over the likely cause of Caesar's epilepsy. Sex was proposed as a cure yet it was also believed to be associated with epilepsy as an after-effect of syphilis. One of the more colourful suggestions of Caesar's epilepsy was that it was a price of his womanising. But the most compelling aetiology centres on Caesar's hereditary predisposition, based on an above-average incidence of the condition in the Julio-Claudian families. Historians have speculated that the sudden unexpected deaths of his father and great-grandfather were the consequence of epilepsy. Caesar's descendants Caligula and Tiberius Claudius were also said to have suffered from epilepsy.

Julius Caesar's seizures were hugely important and directly impacted on at least two significant moments in history and in his life: a perceived slight of the magistrates of the Senate in the period leading up to his assassination; and earlier in the Battle of Thapsus.

The African campaign in the Roman civil war between Caesar and Pompey's armies culminated at the Battle of Thapsus in

46 BC. You know you're on less-than-firm ground when the same historian, Plutarch, gives competing versions of the battle: one in which Caesar is at the head of his army; and the other in which he is ferried from the battleground and is detained after an epileptic attack. What is not disputed is the mayhem that followed the battle.

Several sources suggest that Caesar's epilepsy was a factor, not in determining victory or defeat, but in the fortunes of his vanquished opponents. 'Caesar the Merciful' had a name befitting his reputation for showing mercy in victory. But in some accounts he is depicted as having undergone a dramatic transformation (worthy of Hollywood), turning from merciful to merciless in the aftermath of Thapsus.

In other reports, more in keeping with his character, Caesar is alleged to have suffered an epileptic attack in the midst of the fighting and was stretchered off to a nearby tower to rest and recover. He was not sufficiently conscious to decide on the fate of those remnants of Pompey's army who had escaped but had not committed suicide. Hours later, with his faculties restored, Caesar discovered to his horror that the defeated soldiers' offer to surrender had been spurned. Ten thousand of Pompey's broken army had been massacred by Caesar's rampant legions.

Some critics have argued that this latter version, with the stricken Caesar shocked by the news of the massacre, was concocted to help maintain his reputation, especially in light of his policy of clementia (mercy); and to absolve him of blame for what followed.

A subsequent seizure more than a year later, recorded in Plutarch's *Life of Julius Caesar*, was the source for Shakespeare's drama in which the dictator's epileptic attack foreshadows the tragedy that is about to unfold, with the unheeded warning of his eventual assassination. Shakespeare was aware of *morbus comitialus*, the Roman custom whereby public meetings (the *comitialus*) were abandoned at the first sign of anyone succumbing to epilepsy. An epileptic seizure was deemed to be a bad omen. Shakespeare's play *Julius Caesar* infers that the general was clearly losing his grip.

In the first act, Mark Antony offers Caesar the emperor's crown three times, but Caesar, in the midst of an epileptic attack, does not respond:

CASSIUS: But soft, I pray you. What, did Caesar swoon?

CASCA: He fell down in the marketplace, and foamed at mouth, and was speechless.

BRUTUS: 'Tis very like. He hath the falling sickness.

The 'Falling Sickness', another ancient name for epilepsy, was still in common usage in Elizabethan England. In that first act, Shakespeare dramatised an event that historians had recorded with varying interpretations. On his return to Rome after the civil wars, friends and enemies of Caesar were queuing up to curry favour and flatter him. Plutarch wrote, 'When they had decreed divers honours for [Caesar] in the Senate, the Consuls and Praetors, accompanied by the whole assembly of the Senate, went unto him in the market-place, where he was set by the pulpit for orations, to tell him what honours they had decreed for him in his absence. But he, sitting still in his majesty, disdained to rise up unto them when they came in, as if they had been private men.'

Caesar's perceived contempt for the sycophants and his breach of protocol was viewed as yet more evidence of his arrogance and his dismissal of the powers vested in the Senate. They were unaware that, actually, Caesar had been unable to rise because he'd suffered a seizure.

One of the debilitating and humiliating consequences of an epileptic seizure can be a temporary loss of control of the sphincter muscles around the urethra and anus. Some historians, such as

Dio Cassius, argued that during the attack Caesar had opened his bowels. But the idea that Caesar's alleged contempt of the senate was instead an attempt to disguise the seizure and incontinence seems improbable.

Plutarch relates contemporary reports that Caesar offered his illness as an apologia to 'excuse his folly' for his improper behaviour: 'He imputed it to his disease, saying, that their wits are not perfect which have this disease of the falling evil, when standing on their feet they speak to the common people, but are soon troubled with a trembling of their body, and a sudden dimness and giddiness.'⁴

But Caesar was not immune to the stigma of the condition and is unlikely to have drawn attention to his affliction. The makers of the 1963 film *Cleopatra* allude to this in the scene where Cleopatra (Elizabeth Taylor), peeping through a hole in the wall into Caesar's chamber, observes him having a fit. The other side of the wall is painted with an enormous eye, reflecting Caesar's nervousness about disclosure and the threat of his power being diminished if the public was to learn of his epilepsy.

In any event, alongside the psychological impact, the fit itself would have been physically draining. As Aretaeus wrote, following a seizure the epileptic was 'spiritless and dejected from the shame and suffering of the dreadful malady'. Either way, whether Caesar was shown to be insultingly autocratic or weakened by the malady, the die was cast as far as the conspirators and would-be assassins were concerned in the build-up to the Ides of March.

Whilst retrospective diagnosis of epilepsy in historical figures is always dangerous, the balance of probability suggests Caesar did suffer from epilepsy and that at significant moments those seizures, whether partial, complex (absences) or generalised, led to a temporary loss of his faculties. Historians and physicians down the ages have consistently interpreted this temporary neurological impairment as clouding his judgement or altering his behaviour sufficiently for him, for example, to fail to heed the warnings and to dismiss the guards who might have saved his life.

How difficult must it be to accommodate the notion that there will be periods of absence throughout your life, when you will wake up not only in the presence of strangers but that you might be dependent on them for your protection.

Recently, after another incident J had found herself waking up on a stranger's sofa: 'There was a lady next to me and I looked down and I was wearing an old shirt and some Y-fronts. It was in the early hours and apparently I'd run out of my flat near naked, just in a shirt; and I'd stopped and asked this stranger who was coming back from a night shift if she knew where I could buy biscuits. She took me to her home. I wasn't wearing any underwear and she wanted to preserve my dignity so she found a new pair of Y-fronts that her deceased husband had never worn. A little while later I woke up and she told me what had gone on.'

It was the memory of this post-seizure experience and her past knowledge of the kindness of strangers that got J out of the door in the mornings when she felt timid, when she feared a fit in public. Her past told her that she could count on strangers now and in the future. But there was a caveat: 'I'm really aware of the particular response to me being five foot three and quiet – and I dress quite smartly. I just wonder how different it would be if I was someone else, if I was male or tall or scruffier or intimidating – if I was your brother.'

Epilepsy has changed J's character; she is necessarily more cautious. The condition imposes limitations on life which J has no choice but to accept. 'It's like an unruly beast which I have to bargain with,' she says. 'It's not something that rules my life but I have to negotiate with it.' Prior to the attack on her, J had been a keen cyclist: it had been part of her identity. It struck me that her acceptance of her inability to cycle was akin to the crushing realisation that Christopher had had to accommodate: neither could return to the self they'd been before.

But there were regular reminders of her luck. Recently, after an attack J had been taken to A&E. She was given an MRI scan which evidently confused the medics who huddled round the terminal trying to make sense of it. 'Basically, according to the scan,' says J, 'I shouldn't have been alive. And the medics looked like they were trying to work out how they could tell me that I was dead.'

Colonies of Mercy

By 1990, my brother Christopher was grown up and soon to leave home, but he was still, and would for ever remain, the baby of the family. Months before he did leave, my mother woke from a dream of terrible foreboding. In her dream she was much younger, perhaps thirty, and was in a field watching her children happily at play. Someone whose face she did not see came up behind her and whispered in her ear, 'They shall leave you one by one, until you are all alone.' My mother was terrified that the message was a warning that her children would die before her – perhaps Christopher, whose diagnosis was now confirmed, first as he was the most vulnerable. It took a while for me to persuade her otherwise; that her dream was really a reflection of her own mortality and attendant angst that the parent of a child with disability feels when considering who will care for that dependent child when the parent dies; or more likely it was an expression of the separation anxiety that many mothers feel when the time comes for their children to leave home. Although in the story of epilepsy, for some the leave-taking is the other way around: a version of the Hansel and Gretel story in which the mother abandons the child.

In 1943, Sandy, a four-year-old child, was escorted by her mother to a residential home for children and left there overnight. The next day came and went with no sign of her mother, or the next day, or the next. Her mother never returned. A decade passed and

Sandy, now a teenager, was transferred from the children's home to an epileptic colony for adults on a farm in Chalfont, Buckinghamshire. She has remained there ever since. Her mother never visited. Nobody visited – neither friend nor relative. Sandy's only visitor was her epilepsy. She's now seventy-one; and apart from those first four years she has spent her life in the company of helpers and other people with epilepsy.

There'd been a flicker of disappointment when I'd walked in to interview Sandy at the residence.[1] She had just settled down with her feet up in front of the television. I was clearly not the highlight of her day. Sandy was dependent on the staff. But I was impressed by her pridefulness, the way she put anyone on guard who might be tempted to fuss around her. She declined my help, easing herself from the sofa to the wheelchair which she needed to get around in after an epileptic seizure had left her with a broken knee. As Sandy wheeled herself out of the room the staff backed away like anxious but hopeful parents encouraging their child's first unassisted steps.

Of her arrival at the epileptic colony (still home to a dwindling number of residents but now also a centre of research into epilepsy) more than fifty years ago, Sandy only remembered her unease over the thinness of the curtains in her dormitory that allowed for little privacy. She had no theory about why her mother had abandoned her. In the beginning, yes, she'd been curious but as the seasons passed, the years and the decades, she'd stopped reflecting on it. Memory had crusted over. Sandy hadn't considered it for a very long time, and she waved away my further questions on the topic. She didn't want to think about it.

There had been no let-up in Sandy's seizures over the years; they were so common that she had ceased to mark them, and she could not recall her last seizure when I asked her. Some time ago Sandy had concluded that her epilepsy could not be defeated: it could only be accommodated. Epilepsy might have been the key determining factor of her life, but it need not define her.

The residential care offered to Sandy is a luxury hardly replicated around the world. Even at Chalfont she seems an enigma now. Unlike Sandy, the majority of residents at this former epileptic colony have learning disabilities and severe and frequent seizures requiring them to wear protective helmets to soften their many falls.

Though people with epilepsy are still marginalised by sections of society, their quality of life is much improved from even sixty years ago. Then exposed to the general hostility of the outside world, some people with epilepsy sought refuge and retreat. The Welsh poet Margiad Evans found her self-consciousness about her epilepsy enormously debilitating. In her 1950s autobiography, *A Ray of Darkness*, she sympathised with those whose 'shyness of suffering might make [them] long to enter a colony rather than attempt to lead a private life which is no longer private'.

Even into the twentieth century, one of the biggest problems faced by people with epilepsy was that they didn't fit in, no matter what strand of society they came from. A decade after the Chalfont colony opened, Britain's royal family made the decision to remove Prince John from public scrutiny. From the age of twelve, King George V's youngest son, who suffered from uncontrolled epilepsy, was hidden away and settled with his own household at Wood Farm on the Sandringham Estate. Most were not so fortunate. Unless their family was wealthy enough and willing to care for them, people with epilepsy would find themselves at the mercy of the authorities who confined them to workhouses or their equivalent.

In a journal published in May 1850 Charles Dickens describes a visit to a squalid metropolitan workhouse. 'A Walk in a

Workhouse' sees him enter a processing room (he calls it a 'kind of purgatory') that is filled mostly with 'noisy mad women' and a single sane supervisor. A prettily dressed twenty-three-year-old girl attracts his attention. She is 'of most respectable appearance, and good manners brought in from the house where she had lived as domestic servant on account of being subject to epileptic fits'.[2]

Dickens pities the girl and is scandalised by her plight. She ought not, by rights, to be there. She is not insane but in the company of the mad women (about whom she pathetically complains) she is destined to end up like them. This servant girl's circumstances were not atypical. She would have been better off in that unnamed workhouse if she'd been a thief, caught and jailed. But as a pauper with epilepsy, along with 2,000 other grim souls, she was crammed in to that pestilent and depressing institution.

Workhouses were an attempt to cleanse vagabonds from the streets; to contain and confine them. The first opened in Bristol in 1697, and over the course of the next century their numbers grew quickly.[3] By the time Dickens walked through the door in the unnamed parish of 'St So and So', he could have chosen from over a hundred just like it in England. And in those houses of misery all manner of poor people were thrown together: beggars, waifs, single mothers, the unsupported elderly, the insane and epileptics. Often little distinction was made between these latter two groups. Even as the nineteenth century drew to a close people with epilepsy were still tainted by the notion of madness or demonic possession.

The idea had been centuries in the making; attendant with it many European countries had adopted policies of exclusion and segregation. The workhouse in England and the German *Zuchthaus* had their roots in earlier manifestations as houses of correction. But perhaps Paris offered the most startling example of the limits of the state's tolerance and duty of care.

In 1606, under a parliamentary directive, vagrants were expelled from Paris and discouraged from returning by companies of archers stationed at all the gates to the city. But even under threat they crept back, bred and gave birth to the next generation of poor within the boundary walls. The king was adamant that something had to be done about them. Fifty years after the expulsion the Hôpital Général was established and, by royal decree, hordes of paupers were rounded up and interned in its vast complex of buildings (including the former gunpowder factory, Salpêtrière) until their numbers swelled to 6,000 – 1 per cent of the capital's population.[4] The title '*hôpital*' appeared to be a misnomer. For though it demonstrated a softening of previous attitudes towards the poor and was designed to accommodate them – no matter their age or sex, whether able-bodied or invalid, insane or epileptic – the directors of the institution were given free rein to keep the populace in check 'having for these purposes stakes, irons, prisons and dungeons so much as they deem necessary' with inmates afforded no licence to appeal against their regulations. It would take many decades to shrug off the ugly stains of its past, but from these unpromising beginnings France's premier neuropsychiatric institution would later emerge. Though, as the Hôpital Général evolved into a medical establishment, people with epilepsy continued to be lumped together with the insane, a distinction was drawn at least amongst the fledgling neurologists that its cohort of epileptics might be constituted both from the rational and the insane.

Elsewhere, the growing recognition that people with epilepsy were not mad but in need of social care (for which there was no state provision) was the impetus behind the founding of epileptic 'colonies of mercy'. 'Neglected by man and seemingly forgotten by God' was the verdict of the superintendent of New York State's epileptic colony on the plight of his inmates; his institution was going to correct that oversight.[5]

The epileptics' colony movements in the USA and Britain took their cue from Germany's Bielefeld Institution; as well as from eugenicist thinking on the need to segregate pathogenic elements in society from the more healthy working classes. The varying practices of the epileptic colonies reflected the fact that even amongst philanthropists there were national and cultural prejudices towards the afflicted.

Work was the key driver for the advocates for a colony to be established close to Bielefeld. Its founders were animated by the reluctance of businesses to employ people with epilepsy; not only was it dispiriting and wasteful of human potential but it also perpetuated a culture of prejudice and sanctioned ignorance. Setting up an epileptic colony was hugely important; it would prove to be the most significant development for people with epilepsy in hundreds of years, and the axis on which public perception of them would begin to turn.

Of all the European countries in the nineteenth century, Bismarck's Germany recognised that the huge changes to life wrought by the headlong rush towards industrialisation, as well as the rapid migration of masses of people from the countryside to the towns, needed urgently to be addressed.

Germany was the first country to adopt the principle of compulsory health and accident insurance for its factory workers, and the introduction of pensions in old age or in the event of disability. Nonetheless bands of desperate artisans continued to tramp through the country in search of work; and in the hierarchy of those most likely to be discriminated against, the man or woman suffering from epilepsy was close to the top.[6]

Germany's social experiment began with a focus on people with epilepsy in the district of Bielefeld, a semi-industrial town with an age-old reputation for the production of linen. In the middle of the nineteenth century it became home to a large mechanised spinning mill. And later, over a thousand people worked in its sewing machine repair factory which opened in 1867. But Bielefeld was also in the heart of fertile farmland, an area called the Ravensberger, and in the same year of the factory opening its gates, a small group of concerned citizens determined to find shelter for a handful of men with epilepsy.[7] They purchased a property, renamed Eben-Ezer, which would become the corner-stone of the first 'Evangelic Sanatorium for Epileptics'. Four men moved into the peasant farmhouse in a quiet valley surrounded by beech woods and a hill at the foot of an old turreted castle.

Contemporaneous accounts of the evolution of the Bethel colony (a few miles off the beaten track from Bielefeld) read like a fable, one that starts as a Grimm fairy tale but ends happily – a misty-eyed romance of an idea culminating in a utopian idyll. Typically, somewhere in a distant part of Germany or an adjoining country a young orphan, who develops epilepsy after witnessing his mother being struck by lightning, is dispatched by ancient relatives (too elderly to care for him) with a few rations and the name of Bethel and its pastor sewn into the lining of his coat. He finds his way to the Colony of Mercy, and though Bethel is full to bursting, the colonists make room for one more unfortunate soul. The boy's life is transformed; years later he is even married by the local pastor on the *deel* (threshing floor) and goes on to become a pillar of society.

Such marriage ceremonies would have been conducted by Friedrich von Bodelschwingh, the pastor who became most closely associated with Bethel. Often pictured with a bible in hand as if he was on the witness stand about to take the oath, von Bodelschwingh was quietly charismatic with 'the smile of child-hood' but also a face marked by the extraordinary gravitas of 'a man of centuries'. The son of the former prime minister of Prussia, Pastor Friedrich swapped the grandeur of a Berlin mansion for the basic comforts of Bethel. 'It is remarkable', wrote one admirer, to see him 'with his idiots. How they cling to his love!' The pastor was helped in his ministry and administration by a dedicated team of deacons and deaconesses – the white-capped 'sick nurses, Bible women and messengers of Christ' rolled into one.

After the arrival of the initial gang of four, Bethel expanded rapidly with numerous houses and eventually over a thousand colonists, guided by a simple mission: 'to bind up the broken hearted' and to provide refuge for 'a commonwealth of sufferers'. Those sufferers would be drawn from a cast not only of 'epileptics', but of 'imbeciles', the 'temporarily insane' and those with 'weak nerves'.

Part of the success of Bethel stemmed from the location: the village estate was fringed by the Teutoburgian Forest, providing a natural barrier from the outside world, and a shield from stigma for its colonists. In the overarching ethos at Bethel, 'a fit became merely an unimportant episode in life when it no longer rendered him whom it befell a pariah among his fellows'.[8]

Within a few years of its founding the number of colonists had grown to twenty-five. By 1871 several religious wardens (house parents) had joined the colony. Whilst its intentions had remained modest Bethel did not attract any hostility, but the announcement of plans to start work on a new building for another hundred men with epilepsy provoked outrage amongst locals. However, it seems Elder von Bodelschwingh was also a master of diplomacy. Not only did he assuage fears about the speed of expansion with the promise that he would, as it were, 'run behind the cart and apply the brakes'; but he later established an association, Arbeiterheim, for local, working-class townsfolk whose resentment of the colony's growth was not apparently contradicted by their willingness to sell land to Bethel.

Though supported by subscriptions and donations, Bethel aimed for self-sufficiency and to adhere to the principle of work for each according to his ability: 'If he can only push a wheelbarrow, then he shall have a wheelbarrow to push.' The work ethic (*Arbeitserziehung*) was seen as a tool, an instrument of repair that would not just be physical but spiritual. The colony prided itself also on the range of work it was able to offer the inmates: farming and brickmaking proved profitable, adding to the coffers of the treasury. There was a bakery, and a restaurant in the great hall. The printing office and the book-binding works were much prized. But the pharmacy was especially lucrative. The majority of Bethel's patients took bromide 'as regularly as daily bread'. Prudently, the colony, requiring half a ton of bromide per month, decided to manufacture its own, and by so doing ensured that its colonists received a purer version of the drug than could be found in the big cities, with consequentially fewer signs of 'bromide face' (skin eruptions) that were a common side effect. Bethel even began to export bromide: orders for its outpatient prescriptions were received from beyond the borders of Germany, as far as Sumatra.

At its peak, Bethel attracted ten times the number of applicants that it could accommodate, despite the fact that it subsequently grew quickly from one major house with everyone under the same roof, to several smaller shared houses, each with biblical names: 'Eben-Ezer', of course, was the original. Others included 'Bethlehem' which housed the bakers; and 'little Nazareth' for the carpenters. Expansion also helped redress initial teething problems as the institution was established along the lines of the existing Germanic social order. Inmates paid for their upkeep according to their means – which occasionally led to disputes as it was 'very difficult to provide first- and second-class patients with the comforts for which they paid, without exciting the jealousy of the third-class patients, many of whom are admitted free.'[9]

The upper-class men were eventually housed in 'Hermon' and they went on to provide many of the clerks for the offices and librarians at the colony. 'Bethany' became the epileptic ladies' house, graced with its own 'pleasant garden . . . sitting room, cosy corners and harmonium, of course'. £100 per year entitled the first-class patients to a room of their own. (Second-class accommodation was priced at £50 per annum.)

Sister Laura, the widow of a Prussian general (who by her own admission was 'as tough as shoe leather'), presided over 'Bethany'. Neither she nor the team who oversaw the Colony of Mercy (as it became known) shirked from the notion that involuntary confinement might occasionally be required for some of its inmates. Further up the hill from 'Bethany', 'Bethesda' was reserved for non-epileptic 'ladies of good position and rank' but with weak nerves who needed to be taken in hand. If not then they were surely destined for 'Magdala', the female asylum, 'a place of refuge . . . for women epileptics under temporary insanity'.[10]

One key development that arose from Bethel was that up until its founding no one had really considered the scale of the condition suffered by its inmates. Sympathisers worried about the effect on individuals with epilepsy of seeing others in the throes of a fit. Before their arrival at Bethel, it was argued (because of loss of consciousness during fits) that people with epilepsy would have been unaware of the distressing manifestation of seizures. That argument would prove to be unfounded. Nonetheless Bethel had to fight constantly the pessimism of those who saw no future for people with epilepsy and who agonised over the inward state of the epileptic sufferer because, 'He knows there is an uncanniness about his condition which makes even friends say, "Twere better he were dead."'

Colonists themselves could have been forgiven such morbid thoughts as death regularly drummed on the doors of the village.

The life expectancy from birth for the German population in the period 1891–1900 was just over forty for men and forty-three for women.[11] But at Bethel few reached more than thirty. One correspondent noted, 'The mortuary bell of the colony may be heard five or six times a week.' But its epileptic population does not appear to have been crestfallen by the high mortality rate. Funerals were very well attended, and sermons from the Zion church attested to the belief that death was part of life, and that escape from Babylon warranted not mourning but rather celebration. It was a view borne out by the way colonists recounted to visitors the extraordinary death of one of its pastors who had recently confessed to the congregation that he too suffered from epilepsy. At the end of a day when the pastor had been inexplicably agitated, he'd jumped into a pony trap and set off at quite a lick, furiously whipping the pony as he drove. As the trap rushed through the countryside, the pastor lost control, and when the pony pulled up sharply, he was thrown from the conveyance, hit his head on a rock, suffered a violent seizure and died. Sad though it was the colonists were comforted by the vision of the pastor in the pony trap 'going home, even like Elijah, in a chariot of fire'.[12]

Not only was the Bethel colony touted as a model institution, it also attracted visitors from around the world who left galvanised with plans to realise versions of Bethel in their own countries.[13] In its care of people with epilepsy, England did not compare favourably with Germany. Returning home from an inspiring pilgrimage to Bethel, campaigners fulminated over the startling differences between the two countries. Obviously when one looked at humankind's evolutionary tree the Englishman was on the branch just down from God, but one still had to admit that there were some things that Germany appeared to do better.

Fifty years after Dickens's 'A Walk in a Workhouse', a report by the Local Government Board highlighted that there were more than 600 'sane epileptics' in the workhouses of London alone. Not only was their incarceration inappropriate but such people were also all too often at the mercy of ignorant and malicious workhouse staff. On 2 February 1894, the *Echo*'s headline, 'An Epileptic Pauper Persecuted', spelt out the plight of Anne Farcombe who'd been jailed three times for violent conduct in the workhouse. In court her defence that each time she'd actually been suffering fits was dismissed by workhouse officials who said she'd been 'shamming'. On her fourth imprisonment it was clear there'd been no pretence when she endured a number of fits in jail and the governor subsequently sanctioned her release.

But where liberal critics such as Dickens were appalled by the brutal conditions and forced labour of the workhouses, more conservative Establishment figures decried what they saw as its encouragement of privileged idleness.

Charitable works were never entirely freed from considerations of, and domain assumptions about, class and entitlement in England. The alleviation of the suffering and humiliation of people with epilepsy was subservient to the urgent need to address their blight on civil society. The disorder and other dangers posed by this so-called 'degenerate group' far exceeded the abilities of the poor laws to combat them. England's poor laws were such that vagrants would have to tumble into the gutter before any assistance was offered; and when it came to campaigns to set up homes for the relief of the poor, stray dogs had a greater pull on the heart-strings of the public than vagabond families – whether deserving or undeserving poor made little difference. Nonetheless, as in other countries, the notion of an English colony of mercy emerged from accounts of Bethel by visitors who, inspired by a vision of social Christianity in action, sought an opportunity back home to do charitable work among people with epilepsy.

The groundwork, in some regards, had already been prepared by a new breed of doctor, neurologists, whose patients at the National Hospital for the Paralysed and Epileptic included more than 50 per cent who suffered from epilepsy. The hospital, which opened at Queen Square in London in 1860, quickly established itself as a mecca for neurologists. On 11 April 1892 they gathered in London with the intention of founding an organisation with Bethel as its template. Their timing was fortuitous as others were thinking along similar lines. Fundamentally, the idea for a colony emerged through the convergence of medical enlightenment with social engineering and philanthropic forces in Britain.[14]

Skipping's Farm, a suitable (some even said salubrious) estate was purchased to accommodate in the first instance a group of eighteen men in a remote part of the countryside not far from the village of Chalfont St Peter, Buckinghamshire.[15] Initially the colony was only open to men, in particular those who could afford the 10 shillings fee and demonstrated a willingness to work: accommodating both sexes was considered too problematic; and equally children were barred. On 31 July 1894 the very first colonist, W. Bullock, entered the temporary accommodation, a corrugated-iron building that had been erected close to the eighty-year-old farmhouse. In a letter to the *Polytechnic Magazine*, Mr Bullock remarked on the beauty of the surroundings, and was pleased to note that though a church service was conducted for the Anglican majority, 'respect is paid to the feelings of such Dissenters as myself'. For entertainment the men gathered around a piano each Sunday evening. And finally Bullock expressed his gratitude for his time at the colony:

> Although at intervals I have forced upon me the disagreeable truth that I am still an epileptic, I consider that my health has improved during my stay here. There is about the

vegetables [grown on the farm] a freshness I never tasted in London, while the nearest approach to a fog is a light mist. The soil is loam, with subsoil of gravel and chalk, and we are at an altitude of 400 feet above sea level.

The clue to the aims of the establishment was to be found in its name: the National Society for the Employment of Epileptics (NSEE). Skipping's Farm was a great choice. The young tenant farmer, Mr Sills, remained in the farmhouse and was contracted to help till the land. And in the first instance, the colonists found that the soil was excellent for planting hazel, cherry trees and evergreens. But the neurologists who were represented on the Executive Committee also envisaged that the colony would serve as a research institute; so that from the beginning there was tension at the NSEE over whether Chalfont represented a chance to solve the medical condition of patients or to alleviate their social and economic problems.

The Ladies' Samaritans saw Chalfont primarily as a chance to offer brutalised epileptics a refuge from asylums and jails. Penelope, the lady columnist of the *Western Times, Exeter*, echoing Dickens, believed that 'an epileptic patient is not necessarily a lunatic but many an epileptic has been driven into insanity by enforced association with lunatics'. Fresh air would provide a tonic and work of course would contribute to their upkeep because, as the *Daily News* reported, the general purpose of the colony was to be a 'busy little hive of industry with two sorts of product – the fruits of the earth and manufactured articles for sale'. Such sentiments were in keeping with the tough-minded philanthropists at the NSEE who were guided by the notion of eradicating begging and the abuse of charity through hard graft. Still others, such as the eugenicist Sir James Crichton-Browne, were keen to promote the colony as a means of ensuring that epileptics did not marry. Asked directly by an anxious gentleman supporter whether colony patients would be allowed to marry, the answer that came back from the committee (reassuringly for the gentleman) was a 'firm No!'

All camps, though, were unified by the high-minded ideals hammered out by the neurologists on 11 April 1892: that the colony would serve as 'a home for such epileptic persons as are capable of work but unable to obtain regular employment on account of their liability to fits'. Just how crucial this was and how difficult it might be to achieve was demonstrated a few years later when one of the first teachers at Chalfont (who also happened to suffer from epilepsy) was dismissed because she had a fit during a class.

Whilst the founders courted benefactors, they were also conscious of the unfortunate fact that the local population still clung to prejudices about epilepsy (believing that 'persons afflicted were dangerous lunatics'). The staff were at pains not to draw attention to the new inhabitants of Skipping's Farm. Class, they were to learn, was no barrier to ignorance. Early on, a curtain-twitching neighbour whose property overlooked the settlement complained that he'd witnessed a colonist having a seizure. The committee earnestly debated his complaint and concluded that it was unfounded. The hedge was deemed high enough but, they conceded, perhaps it needed a little thickening in places.

Discretion was to be the watchword at Chalfont. Yet it was not always clear whom the discretion was intended to benefit, especially when it was extended to masking the identity of new arrivals. On processing and admission to the institution the colonists' names were removed from the records: they were identified only by a number.

The curtain twitchers of Chalfont or those scrambling up step-ladders to peep over hedges in disgust appear to have been in a minority. The local population's response was relatively sanguine, at least compared to the blood-boiling fulminations of residents of other affluent areas who were traumatised by the prospect of having undesirable colonists as neighbours. In 1907, *The Times* reported, regarding the problem of where to house people with epilepsy, that the 'can' had not just been 'kicked up the street' from one squalid London borough to the next but had been booted into the green pastures of the Home Counties, despoiling formerly desirable areas such as Epsom.

Lord Rosebery, the former prime minister, was particularly incensed that not only was the council accommodating lunatics in palatial asylums (paid for by the poor ratepayer) but epileptics too were adding to the 'flood of unhealthy, insanitary and mentally decayed persons'. It was enough to cause the 5th Earl of Rosebery to abandon the Durdans, the Epsom country estate which until recently had been his favourite of his various homes.[16]

Chalfont escaped such outpourings of grievance. From its inception Skipping's Farm and its colonists met with favourable if patronising reviews from newspapers throughout the country. The *Yorkshire Herald* noted approvingly that 'a spirit of altruism' was fostered among the inmates that 'reduced the tendency to morbid introspection and irritability to which victims of the falling sickness are prone'. *The Times* also applauded from the sidelines but assured its readers that 'the purchase of drink is strictly forbidden under pain of instant dismissal'.[17]

But though it was a retreat and haven for people with epilepsy, Chalfont was not free from the tensions, class and sexual, that ran through society outside: indeed it was a microcosm of English society. At either end of the spectrum were the patients and nursing staff. The patients were largely working class; the nurses were expected to be 'gentlewomen' (actual nursing qualifications were only necessary for the sisters and matrons); and the gardeners and artisans were somewhere in between.

There was to be no fraternising between the classes and especially between the sexes. When, for instance, it was brought to the attention of the committee that a nursing sister had taken leave of her senses and, in breach of the unspoken social mores of the time, had gone walking after 10 p.m. with the tenant farmer, Mr Sills, she was immediately dismissed.[18]

The biggest contention in the colony, however, was whether Chalfont should be primarily a medical or social institution – whether a medical superintendent should exert supreme control over the colony's patients and staff. Sir James Crichton-Browne, for one, thought the question absurd because the 'dominant fact [was that] epilepsy and every detail of its management must have reference to the characteristics of the disease'. Sir James believed that one should no more consider an epileptic colony without a medical superintendent than one would countenance a public school without a headmaster.[19]

Doctors of Crighton-Browne's persuasion looked on with envy at the free rein given to medical supervisors on the other side of the Atlantic. In America, New York State opened its first settlement, the Craig colony near Sonyea, in 1896. Built on communal land acquired from the Shakers (whose belief in celibacy ensured their extinction), the colony was ten times the acreage of Skipping's Farm and expected to cater for 500 patients.

Craig colony boldly stated its mission to segregate and treat epileptics exclusively. It separated the sexes and divided patients into three classes: curable, incurable and violent. As a matter of principle 'no insane or mentally retarded epileptics would be admitted since their behaviour would interfere with epileptics of normal intelligence'. Dr William Phillip Spratling oversaw the running of the institution (having spent the spring of 1892 at Bethel colony). Spratling was a powerful advocate for the colony but his attempts to explain in layman's terms the mental state of his charges sometimes risked sowing confusion. 'In all cases, scientifically or even clinically speaking,' he told one group of investigators, 'epileptics border on the insane, only in one case the mental unsoundness is continuous, and in the other periodic.'[20] By temporary or periodic insanity, Spratling was referring to the seizure state when people were not fully in control of their faculties. Such people were candidates for Craig colony.

The archetypal prospective colonist, it was recognised, found himself in an invidious position in the nineteenth century. Marginalised from an early age, noted the physician Frederick Petersen, he was likely to be expelled from school, to discover in adulthood that it was almost impossible to find employment, and to be refused admission to general hospitals. Finally, cast adrift from respectable society, like his counterpart in England, he'd end his days locked up in an insane asylum because there was no alternative place of safety for him.

Interviewed by the *New York Times* about the 'Interesting Village of Sonyea where Afflicted are Cared For', Dr Spratling extolled the notion that people with epilepsy, who'd been left to grow idle and ignorant, might find salvation in work. Agriculture was the staple industry at the Craig colony. And championing the virtues of labour, Spratling noted a trebling of the number of fits amongst the patients on rainy days when agricultural work could not be done. He also pointed out that the greatest threat to the colony came from the instance of one epileptic suffering a seizure that led to mass seizures among the other inmates: 'When one is taken with a fit the whole number about him are apt to fall at once, due to excitement.'[21]

In this regard, the superintendent at Craig colony echoed a number of physicians and other self-appointed specialists on both sides of the Atlantic; men such as John Townsend Trench and Jean-Martin Charcot. In Dublin, Townsend Trench, an amateur architect and chairman of the Poor Laws Guardians for Ireland, ran a private clinic for people with epilepsy, and maintained that epilepsy was contagious; that 'the disease is telegraphed from one epileptic to another' as is 'hysteria among women'.²² And in Paris at the Salpêtrière institution, the leading neurologist Charcot argued vehemently that patients with epilepsy should be kept apart from his insane patients because the sight of a person in the throes of an epileptic seizure might induce the same in his mentally ill patients.

This mimetic possibility was reason enough for some to worry over the wisdom of bringing people with epilepsy together – whether in colonies or insane asylums. But if Spratling was sending out mixed and confusing signals, it was because as an administrator, in a bid to secure funds, he had to navigate a treacherous path between discretion and persuasion. At times, whether addressing newspapermen or possible benefactors, he spoke clinically, with a physician's candour, characterising people with epilepsy admitted to the colony as 'irritable, fault finding, exacting, often violent, destructive and dangerous'. And by way of explanation, if anyone doubted it was so, Dr Spratling simply stated that 'this must be the case in a disease that so disastrously affects the brain'.

There is a school of thought in public relations that holds that nothing is more efficacious to your cause than the introduction of fear. In pointing out the dangers posed by people with epilepsy Spratling was flagging up the great service that his institution was providing to society.

Under Dr Spratling's watch Craig colony implemented basic standards of care for people with epilepsy. Once admitted, they would only be discharged from the colony after they'd been free from seizures for two years. Those who developed insanity during their stay would be removed, not to a poorhouse but to an insane asylum run by the state. The poor were not excluded from Craig colony. Financial assistance from the state would secure them a place. But there was one caveat: any such colonists who died at the colony would have to undergo a mandatory autopsy.

Craig colony's huge population allowed Dr Spratling and his colleagues to begin to conduct research and longitudinal studies; to investigate, for instance, the biochemical aetiology of generalised seizures, and also the high rate of premature death of people with epilepsy as had been noted in Bethel.

Unlike his counterparts in England, Spratling and his team of medics resided in the grounds of the colony. Spratling moved his family into an attractive two-storey house with a large veranda which was put to great use during the summer. Conversely, though the colony was a haven for the colonists, it also meant that those who worked there, notwithstanding the branch line to the local railway station, were as cut off from mainstream society as the previous occupants, Shakers who'd been attracted by the location's remoteness. Despite Spratling's wife's complaint about the isolation she and their children felt there, the medical superintendent remained at its helm for fifteen years and oversaw its expansion. According to a 1902 report in the *New York Times*, the Craig colony then accommodated a thousand souls but such was the demand and the length of the waiting list that extra funds were needed so that the intake might be doubled. The colony secured its future through state funding, the munificence of a handful of wealthy donors and public subscription. At its peak in 1939 the colony would become home to more than 2,500 people with epilepsy.

The epileptic colonies were often reported on and championed as benign institutions, founded on a bedrock of altruism. But enlightened self-interest could also have a darker side. In some respects, a number of colonies were just as much dumping grounds as the workhouses that had preceded them. They were places where unwanted and embarrassing epileptic relatives could be kept out of sight; and where, occasionally, the vulnerable colonists might be preyed on.

Individual transgressions by staff paled beside the systematic abuse of people with epilepsy that was sanctioned in the 1920s by a number of countries including Germany and the USA. In several states in the USA, experiments in social engineering were conducted away from prying eyes – as was later evident, for example, at the notorious Lynchburg colony for Epileptics in Virginia. Lynchburg opened in 1910 but within a few years its conviction of the need to separate sane epileptics from other groups began to unravel. Its change of name to include 'Feeble Minded' in the title of the institution reflected a broadening of its remit.[23] The result (inadvertent or not) was to re-establish the connection between epilepsy and insanity.

The growth of the epileptic colony movement had coincided with the rise of eugenicist theories. At the end of the nineteenth century debates around mental hygiene and social engineering began to move from public soapboxes at speakers' corners to county halls and led eventually to legislation restricting people with epilepsy from marriage. In 1895 Connecticut passed a law which made it a criminal offence for epileptic patients to marry or to cohabit as spouses if the wife was younger than forty-five (and therefore still of childbearing age). Sixteen other states followed suit with laws forbidding marriage for people with epilepsy.

Eugenicists, such as the leading advocates Dr and Mrs Davenport, believed that they were working for the good of humanity to 'urge that human bloodlines be relieved of the worst things, that these worst lines be cut off as much as possible'.[24] No matter the advances made in the understanding of epilepsy and the improvements to the quality of the colonists' lives, the domain assumptions remained that people with epilepsy formed part of a deranged and defective class.

Some argued that legal sanctions against marriage were no guarantee of compliance, and that people with epilepsy along with insane or feeble-minded persons would remain a burden on society. More strident eugenicists demanded earlier state intervention, advancing the logic that if no more epileptics were born, then there wouldn't be any need for laws censuring their marriage. Epileptic colonies seemed the obvious place to start. At the turn of the twentieth century a number of states including California and Idaho passed laws permitting forced sterilisation. The medical superintendent of Virginia's Lynchburg colony, Dr John H. Bell, whom eugenicists were to find an ardent sympathiser, was the first to test the legal principle with one of its inmates, Carrie Buck. The 1927 Supreme Court case of *Buck v. Bell* centred on whether the twenty-one-year-old, who was deemed feeble-minded along with her daughter and mother, should be allowed to give birth once more.[25]

In a ruling chiselled in evangelical certainty, the Supreme Court's Justice Wendell Holmes argued, 'It is better for all the world if, instead of waiting to execute degenerate offspring for crime, or let them starve for their imbecility, society can prevent those who are manifestly unfit from continuing their kind. Three generations of imbeciles are enough.'

In the same way that it was a civic duty for the population to consent to vaccination against smallpox for the common good, argued Wendell Holmes, so too should people with known genetic defects such as epilepsy – who already 'sap the strength of the state' – be prepared to make the sacrifice of sterilisation to ensure a fitter society.

Residents at epileptic colonies were to find subsequently that institutions once advertised as places of safety had become traps, clearing houses where virile men and fecund women were rendered infertile. Men such as Dr Bell cast themselves as pioneering social scientists burdened with a task of necessary inhumanity. The surgeons might make the case for sterilisation readily to themselves, but it would prove more difficult to explain to non-consenting patients. Even though they were state sanctioned, the surgical procedures were often carried out under deception.

Soon after the Supreme Court ruling, as Carrie Buck would later recall, staff at the Lynchburg colony told her they were concerned about her appendix, and that they'd have to carry out an urgent operation to remove it before it ruptured. For the next fifty years, until she was tracked down by a researcher in 1979, Carrie Buck remained ignorant of the real purpose of the surgery: to cut and tie her fallopian tubes.[26]

The subjective classification 'feeble minded' inevitably led to people with epilepsy at Lynchburg and other colonies being caught up in the frenzy of involuntary sterilisations that swept through the USA, as more and more states emboldened by the Supreme Court ruling enacted similar laws. In the intervening years (between 1927 and 1979) over 8,000 men and women were subject to enforced sterilisation in the state of Virginia, and tens of thousands throughout the USA.

But the USA was not alone in the coarsening of its attitude towards the inmates of its epileptic colonies. In Germany, the generosity of spirit and elevated sense of a duty of care towards the most vulnerable sections of society as exemplified by Friedrich von Bodelschwingh evaporated in the aftermath of the seismic defeat of the First World War and the stultifying terms of reparations imposed on it by the victorious allies. To some resentful Germans it was galling that whilst the best of its youth had perished in the trenches, the country was left with an unproductive class of degenerates whose needs were a luxury it could ill afford. Such dark and forbidding thoughts even found expression within the grounds of the Bethel colony.

Following the death of Bethel's superintendent in 1910 his son had assumed the directorship. Towards the end of the First World War Friedrich von Bodelschwingh Jr estimated that more than 300 colonists at Bethel were dying each year from starvation. The privations of Bethel mirrored what was happening throughout the nation; and in that climate of desperation von Bodelschwingh (who a decade later in 1933 would find himself as the religious figurehead in the primary position of Reich bishop designate) began to entertain thoughts which, while stopping short of euthanasia for Germany's more feeble-minded population, flirted with the lesser evil of enforced sterilisation. Come crunch time, though, during the ascendancy of Hitler's National Socialist Party and the introduction of its pathological eugenicist laws von Bodelschwingh recovered his moral compass: he defied the Nazis and let them know that he would rather die with his colonists than let any one of them be carted off to destinations from which there was no return.

The eugenics movement and the notion of selective breeding may have begun in England with Francis Galton (who coined the term 'eugenics') but it did not take root and failed to thrive there. British epileptic colonies escaped the horrors of any systematic state-sanctioned abuse. But like many institutions that cared for the vulnerable they also attracted some workers who would prey on them. In true British tradition such transgressions were usually dealt with tactfully. In 1909 a favoured attendant at Chalfont left in disgrace following 'affectionate and indiscreet behaviour' towards some of the boys at the colony. The terms of his dismissal included payment of his £50 passage to Australia on the understanding that no claims would subsequently be made against the colony.[27]

Leafing through the archives at Chalfont, over the decades one comes across a scattering of reports and allegations: a male attendant interfering with boys: 'He had a go with some of the lads – a prod or a quick lift of their privates'; a closet homo-sexual attendant attempting to seduce another: 'What's wrong can't you take a bit of fun?'; sexual relations between a male attendant and a nursing sister who turned a blind eye to the theft of colonists' clothes (including two new pairs of pyjamas and a worn silk shirt): 'I [the sister] let him steal them because he [the attendant] made love to me repeatedly.'[28] These reports are countered, however, by the accounts of the quiet professionalism of the staff and the appreciation of them by residents such as Sandy for whom Chalfont had been the only home she can recall.

Pat Gutsell always knew she had a sister somewhere who was sent away as a child but never spoken of. 'It was all hush-hush,' says Pat. 'I imagined she'd been taken to the woods like something out of Hansel and Gretel and left there.' Pat's parents separated during her childhood. Her mother took custody of her; her father left home taking Pat's brother with him. She had no memory of her sister Sandy, who'd been taken away when Pat was only eighteen months old. One of the few facts known to Pat was that her sister had epilepsy, and that the condition ran through several genera-tions of the family. Her father, an austere man, had epilepsy as did her brother who had died in his thirties following a seizure. Pat's mother never spoke of the missing sister and discouraged any mention of her. But after her mother's death Pat set about trying to locate her sister. Over the years, at family gatherings she'd occasionally overheard the name Chalfont whispered. It was enough of a clue.[29]

In 2008, fifty-five years after she first arrived at Chalfont, Sandy had an unexpected visitor. Her sister, Pat, walked out of the shrouded past and back into her life.

Anger in the Minds of Gods

The nineteenth century saw the emergence of a new discipline, neuroscience. More than anything that had gone before, this new science and in particular neurology dramatically changed the perception of epilepsy. At last people with the condition were able to circumvent their usual destination, the lunatic asylums with the alienists who worked there, and instead enter voluntarily into the care of neurologists.

It was an age of exploration, marked by gentleman scientists who brought with them a passion for the discipline that ranged from the amateur enthusiast to the zealot. Though neuroscientists skewered previously held popular notions about epilepsy of demonic possession and other superstitions, battle still raged over the classification of some epileptic seizures. Were they the result of a pathology in the brain or the consequences of a psychological disturbance, of hysteria?

Chief among the neurologists were two pioneers who exemplified the great difficulty of establishing, even amongst physicians, a consensus about epilepsy: an Englishman, John Hughlings Jackson, and Jean-Martin Charcot from France – the former a retiring intellectual; the latter a scientist showman who choreographed medical demonstrations more suited to the circus than the lecture hall.

In their differing approaches, both men also revealed the symbiotic relationship between patients and doctors. In the 1800s, dozens of doctors from a variety of disciplines became famous through a number of discoveries only made possible by working with and on patients. People with epilepsy would eventually be the beneficiaries of neuroscience. But the immediate rewards were not always so obvious. There was a price to be paid for medical advance. Patients were very much the subject of experiments, and of the necessary inhumanity of physicians and surgeons honing their skills for the benefit of future generations. Ultimately, their fates were determined by doctors – some of whom exhibited the kind of extreme arrogance once the preserve of the gods.

A teaching hospital is a human freak show presided over by ringmasters with white coats and stethoscopes instead of red coat-tails and bullwhips. Our tutor informed us of this fact, chuckling as he spoke, on our first day at medical school. Our futures were dependent on these medical oddities, he explained, and luckily, we had chosen well because the sick would always be with us.

Over time, it seemed to me that all patients admitted to the teaching hospital – including those with epilepsy – entered into a rarely spoken-of pact. Their expert treatment at the hands of the best and brightest doctors that such institutions attract came at a price: patients were obliged to expose themselves to all and sundry, especially the hapless medical students. It was, however, an improvement on the century before. The expert treatment on offer to sufferers of epilepsy in the early part of the nineteenth century included crude experimental failures, amounting to little more than bloodletting.

Our hospital, the London, clad in the gloom of a Dickensian building, had not quite managed to escape the nineteenth century. It had a formidable reputation and though its setting, Whitechapel, was far from glamorous, the brutal workhouse-like architecture of the hospital and medical school was a match for the location and clientele who seemed to have stepped out from a series of etchings by Hogarth. Prior to my arrival, I knew just two things about Whitechapel: first, that the hospital – its most significant land-mark – had, a hundred years earlier, served as a refuge for the pitifully deformed Elephant Man; and second, that it was an unfortunate square to land on when playing the board game Monopoly. I didn't appreciate then the extent to which members of its staff had been central to the story of the evolution of neuro-science and the understanding of epilepsy.

The area was scarred with rubble, barbed wire and condemned buildings. The population was poor. But, as our tutors constantly reminded us, we were privileged: our patients were rich in pathology. It took a while to work out the nature of our connec-tion with the patients. Did we need them more than they needed us or did we both need each other equally? Was it a symbiotic or parasitic relationship? Often our youth and inexperience betrayed us. Having no conception of catatonia, for example, we'd be impa-tient with men who after trekking to the hospital wilfully refused, it seemed, to take the final steps to the reception desk; in A&E we tried our best not to be entertained by the florid schizophrenic or the toothless drunken diabetic who inverted the cigarette to smoke it inside his mouth; and on the neurological wards, unpre-pared, we struggled when witnessing a fit to resist the urge to avert our gaze. Images of student doctors from the century before suggest that they were both more mature and more considerate than us, but I doubt this was really the case. Ultimately, patients were both repulsive and intriguing; but it was impossible to push away the thought that they, the patients, belonged to another class or species, separate from us.

Doctor–patient relations may have evolved with different sets of protocols over the centuries since the London Hospital had opened, but the contract remained the same – the patient at the

London was a volunteer, a tool in the service of teaching. I could see how people such as Christopher, who had inherited something of the Jamaican meme of suspicion about becoming an unwitting guinea pig in medical research, and who did not readily sign up to the unspoken agreement, would be something of a challenge, if not irritation, for medics.

One curious consequence of my brother's diagnosis was that I began to associate any unexpected ringing of the telephone with the news of him having had yet another seizure. Somewhere along the line Christopher's fits had begun to follow a pattern: they were irregularly regular; they could occur on any given day, but when they did arrive it was increasingly between 3 a.m. and 5 a.m. In the autumn of 2000 the phone rang at an unusually late hour. I steeled myself to answer it. A young man with a clipped, slightly hesitant, stuttering voice came on the line. He announced himself as an A&E registrar at Bart's hospital and he wanted to know if I was related to Christopher Grant. Though guarded his speech was also searching: 'He, he says you're his brother. A-are you his brother?'

'Yes. Is he all right?'

The doctor said Christopher was a bit bashed about. 'Still recognisable, though,' he laughed. They'd patched him up. But when I calculated that it'd be about twenty minutes before I could come and get him, the registrar suggested that it wouldn't be necessary because my brother was behaving very oddly and he, the doctor, was really only ringing as a matter of courtesy to inform me that they were about to section him.

'What? What are you talking about?'

'It's n-not a decision we'd take lightly,' he said.

I was expecting more but the doctor, perhaps wary of my tone and the threat of exclamations in my subsequent silence, did not risk adding anything else. I suppose my silence was the fallout from shock and from the looming sense of an injustice. I'd witnessed the same delayed reaction in children before.

As a student I'd noticed when injecting children with a vaccine how they seemed to accept the needle piercing their skin; it was often only afterwards, once the needle was removed, that they'd start to scream. For a moment now I feared *I* might cry. And then, bizarrely, I heard myself screaming at the poor doctor that my brother was not mentally ill but epileptic. Did he not understand the difference? The registrar's speech was as faltering as a car engine failing fully to crank into life. I didn't wait for his answer to arrive, but slammed down the phone, ran out, hailed a taxi and rushed to the hospital.

Behind one of the curtained A&E booths, my brother lounged on his side on a hospital trolley. As usual his nonchalance gently mocked my sense of urgency; made my emotions seem fraudulent. He'd been joking and teasing with a couple of the nurses and I was pleased to see that they treated him with a kind of efficient tenderness. It took less effort than I had imagined persuading the medical team to reverse their decision to detain Christopher on a psychiatric ward. Perhaps the decision hadn't really been made. But before we left, the young registrar, whose stuttering now warmed me to him (what trials he must have undergone when presenting histories on highly charged and unforgiving ward rounds), stepped out from another curtained bay and blocked our path.

His pinstriped suit was more of a surprise than the mustard-coloured tie – a muted attempt at flamboyance that I'd seen before in ambitious registrars considered consultants-in-waiting. I wanted to apologise for our earlier intemperate phone call – maybe he did as well – but the moment was slipping away. The opportunity passed and then it became impossible. I avoided his eyes; he avoided mine. Instead his gaze fastened on Christopher. His stutter still betrayed him as he warned my brother gravely that though he was free to go now, next time he would not be so fortunate. I felt a tang of disapproval in his voice, and sensed that the doctor was really addressing me. We might have been a married couple at the tail end of an argument over how to reprimand an aberrant child. The disagreement had escalated beyond its original source to expose tensions and flaws in the relationship that had hitherto remained tactfully unspoken. 'Next time,' he repeated, 'you might not be so lucky.'

As was his way at such moments, Christopher rolled out his smile – the one that suggested either that he was about to distance himself from whatever was going on and embark on an internal migration or that he was now in possession of a delicious secret that would remain unshared. But there was also pity in that smile for the poor, exasperated medic. I suspect that to my brother the registrar was about as threatening as a traffic policeman cautioning him but not issuing a ticket.

Increasingly, when he'd had a fit in public and been brought to the emergency unit of a hospital, Christopher seemed resigned to (or determined on) an outcome based on chance; as if he had no influence on it. He offered no assistance to doctors ignorant of his epileptic background but stood back and watched (stoical and amused, a spectator to his own unravelling future) the medics' fumbling attempts to reach a diagnosis. There was not much fun to be had from epilepsy. But there was real enjoyment, apparently, in tying up the doctors in Houdini-like ropes of medical history that only he could cut off, if he so wished.

Notwithstanding the part he'd played in this mischievous tendency towards obfuscation that had contributed to the misunderstanding with the Bart's A&E staff, Christopher *had* been lucky. If he'd had the misfortune of being born earlier on in the previous century, he'd have found that physicians made little distinction between epilepsy and madness.

Much of the nineteenth century was preserved at the London Hospital medical school – not only in the museum artefacts of the Elephant Man (his oversized cap and knotted, gnarled femur bone) but in the heavily Gothic wooden decor and cavernous interior of the main building. You could never fully grasp the topography of the place. There were parts of the building which seemed out of bounds, none more so than the dean's office. The corridor that led to it was lined by a photo gallery of his predecessors and other eminent physicians from the London Hospital's hall of fame. First amongst these lions of the profession was a man generally acknowledged as an important pioneer of English neurology, John Hughlings Jackson, an austere-looking Yorkshireman, with a stiff, grey beard and penetrating eyes.[1]

Both Jackson and Charcot prided themselves on diagnosis through the power of intense observation, and both were championed by their peers as the founding fathers of neurology. But it was perhaps the first brain operation on a patient with epilepsy (by a junior colleague of Hughlings Jackson, a young surgeon and vivisectionist) which loosened the stone that led to the nineteenth-century avalanche of interest in determining the origins of epilepsy and its scientific treatment.

On entering the operating theatre, every fledgling surgeon is quickly introduced to the surgical practice and tradition: 'See one. Do one. Teach one.' But what if you have never seen the operation? What if you are one of the first, pioneering brain surgeons confronted with a patient whose cranium you now have to open? What then?

This is precisely the position Victor Alexander Horsley found himself in on 26 May 1886 at London's Queen Square – the site of the country's National Hospital for the Relief and Cure of the Paralysed and the Epileptic.

The National was a voluntary institution paid for by donation and subscription. The idea for the hospital had been dreamt up by campaigning siblings, Edward Chandler and his sisters, Johanna and Louisa, who'd never married and, in lieu of families, had devoted their adult lives to good deeds. The Chandlers had been particularly scandalised by the pitiful plight of people with paralysis and others with epilepsy who were routinely turned away from the wards of general hospitals. Was the cause of such people so hopeless? Why had they been abandoned to their fate? Why such anger in the minds of gods? By their own example (making and selling delicate ornaments to raise funds) and then through newspaper appeals, the persuasive siblings loosened the purse strings of other high-minded Victorians. The Lord Mayor lined up in support as did newspapers such as the *Daily Telegraph*, shaming its readers with a simple question framed in language that highlighted an everyday prejudice: 'Who among the epileptic abortions of our pavements ever received the slightest aid in his malady?'[2]

Louisa Chandler was never to see the results of her labour; she died in 1859, but the following year, Johanna oversaw the opening of the world's first specialist hospital devoted to neurological complaints – a philanthropic institution that would transform the future, preordained it seemed, of people with epilepsy. The siblings' selflessness may have been inspiring (the senior staff who devoted one day a week to the hospital did so without a salary) but such was the prestige of working there that competition for the few posts was fierce. One physician allegedly offered a gift of £1,000 to the hospital on condition that he was appointed to the staff.[3]

The National Hospital began modestly with ten beds. Within a few years, though, it had acquired an 'electrical' treatment room offering electrotherapy. An enormous cylindrical machine with a Muirhead battery occupied most of that room and provided static electricity for the then novel treatment of paralysis. The electrical room, the source of some pride for the National, was unique in English hospitals – a sign of its modernity and its embracing of the latest scientific understanding.[4] Of the treatments available at the new hospital, electrotherapeutics was the most invasive. Neurosurgery had never been attempted at the National. Up until Horsley's arrival there had been no designated operating theatre. In the nineteenth century, the prognosis for recovery post-operatively even from general surgery was not encouraging. For example, the mortality rate among those undergoing surgical procedures for compound fractures was more than 50 per cent. Even if a patient survived the operation, very often infection and sepsis finished them off.

In 1886, no hospital in Britain yet boasted specialism in surgery. At the time, all surgeons fell under a general banner, and subscribed to the widespread belief that when it came to the brain, medical surgery had reached the outer limits of what was possible. As the distinguished surgeon John Eric Erichsen argued, 'There cannot always be fresh fields of conquest by the knife . . . the brain will be forever shut from the intrusion of the wise and humane surgeon.'[5]

In the day room that Horsley converted into a makeshift operating theatre, observers would have to peer through a yellowing mist of carbolic spray (developed by Joseph Lister) that fumigated the room; they'd also have to adhere to Horsley's strict code: 'loud talking and coughing were strictly forbidden, great stress being laid on the danger of wound infection by contamination in this way'.[6]

Traditionally, operating theatres had not been aseptic, hygienic environments. Lister's germ theory, which placed an emphasis on the cleanliness of surgeons' hands and instruments, had made him famous; though the merits of his antisepsis were yet to be universally appreciated, especially by London surgeons jealous of their Scottish counterparts.

But even the originator of antisepsis dismissed the cleanliness of wards as a sideshow; Lister was not alone amongst surgeons in dressing for theatre in an old frock coat 'stiff and glazed with blood' – a proud index of his years of accumulated experience.[7]

Victor Horsley by contrast embraced both asepsis and antisepsis. The twenty-nine-year-old surgeon's notes on that first operation record how fastidiously the head of his patient was shaved, cleaned and then covered with lint soaked in a 1-in-20 solution of carbolic acid before proceeding.[8]

A decade-old injury to the patient's skull indicated the general area of the lesion in the brain. But the pugnacious and patrician Horsley's unbridled confidence and ambidextrous use of scalpel and other surgical instruments would count for nothing if he did not know precisely where to make the incision.

Horsley could not rely on X-rays (they had not yet been discovered) but he wasn't working entirely in the dark. His colleagues at the National Hospital included Hughlings Jackson, William Gowers and David Ferrier. The latter physiologist's live experiments on animal nervous systems had enabled a rudimentary mapping of the brain. Ferrier's skill in roughly localising the regions of the brain that corresponded with movement and sensory perception was matched by physicians such as Gowers and Hughlings Jackson who through careful taking of medical histories (with an emphasis on signs and symptoms), were able to highlight those areas of abnormal activity in the brain that they believed led to seizures.

Horsley's patient was a twenty-two-year-old man, James B, who had suffered a terrible head injury as a child when he'd been run over by a carriage and left with a fractured skull. Fragments of bone had been removed and the wound eventually healed. But from the age of fifteen the boy had begun having intermittent fits.

The fits had worsened over the years. Prior to his arrival at the National Hospital, James B had suffered an astonishing number of uncontrolled seizures. In two weeks alone he'd endured 3,000 fits. The seizures 'occurred in batches', starting in the right leg and extending to the right hand and arm before moving on to the face, 'followed by turning of the head and eyes to the right'.

During the operation Horsley cut and sawed into the skull, pulled back a flap of the cranium to get through the dura mater into the brain and found and removed a sliver of scar tissue (3 × 2 centimetres) that had formed over the initial childhood wound. Although post-operatively James B experienced some partial motor and sensory paralysis, this gradually improved and up until the time Horsley came to publish the results in the *British Medical Journal* a few months later, the patient had been free from the seizures that had plagued him for the last seven years – this notwithstanding that the very act of surgery creates trauma, so that the surgical excision of the original scar tissue on the brain would likely have resulted in another scar to take its place.

With the corrective surgery Horsley determined not only the degree of accuracy of his and Ferrier's experiments to match regions of the brain to motor and sensory function but also the validity of Hughlings Jackson's theory that seizures were caused by an excessive discharge of electrical activity in certain discrete parts (foci) of the cortex.

No further longitudinal study of James B has been found to measure whether he benefited in the long term from the surgery. But certainly other sufferers of epilepsy were beneficiaries. For that they had to thank not only their predecessors who were subject to the pioneering experimental surgery but also animals.

Five years earlier, in 1881, David Ferrier had been summoned before the courts to answer the charge that he had broken the law by continuing to experiment on conscious monkeys instead of killing them before the anaesthesia had worn off. Ferrier's prosecution galvanised the world of science, including figures such as Charles Darwin who voiced his support; whilst the *British Medical Journal* defended Ferrier, citing the case of numerous patients suffering from epilepsy whose treatment and improvement were largely owed to the increased understanding of the working of the brain brought about through employing monkeys as surrogates in clinical trials.[9]

Although the culture at the National Hospital was collegiate, the science of neurology was far from exact and the necessarily speculative nature of the work in this burgeoning discipline often led to conflict. Apart from the inevitable teething problems at the hospital there were stresses and strains in the relationships between these forceful neurologists. In particular, the arguments ranged over whether and when surgery was advisable; as Horsley was to suggest tersely later in his career, 'So long as our powers of diagnosis remain as they are, so long will the vulgar error of regarding surgical treatment as a *dernier ressort* be committed.' In one noted exchange, Horsley and Gowers clashed over a patient whom Gowers, the physician, was handing over to Horsley for surgery. They argued over the precise location of the pathology in the patient's brain, and therefore where the incision in the skull should be made. There was no adjudicator but since it was agreed that surgery was needed, the surgeon, Horsley, assumed primacy: he would have the final say. The argument was not resolved, only deferred. The operation went ahead. The patient died but the hospital board was relieved to report that the autopsy revealed that the dead man had had more than one lesion: both Gowers and Horsley were vindicated. Neither man was at fault. Their professional integrity was satisfied in an honourable draw.[10]

Often the patient is lost in these early accounts of the growth of neurology; the focus is on medical advancement, and the patient is the means to it: his body provides the pathway to enlightenment. Nonetheless, the limits of the surgery were exposed in these early days. How much of the brain would need to be removed for the surgeon to be sure that he'd excised the lot; that no pathology was left behind to resurface at a later date? That surety was still twenty years away, and would only be substantially improved with the development of electroencephalography in the 1930s. Until then the surgeon was little more than in the position of the average batsman whose technique is best described as 'slog-and-hope'; either you hit the boundary for a four or six or you are bowled out for a duck by the first ball.

Horsley's technique evolved through his experiments with animals. But he too would have acknowledged that at this early stage in neurosurgery he was experimenting on human beings as well. His courage and skill were never in doubt. But Horsley's speed when operating sometimes alarmed onlookers – amongst them Harvey Cushing. As described in Cushing's biography, the visiting American neurologist once accompanied Horsley on a home visit where surgery was to be performed:

After sterilising the instruments in Horsley's house and packing them in a towel, [they] went to a well-appointed West End mansion. Horsley dashed upstairs, had his patient under ether in five minutes, and was operating fifteen minutes [later], made a great hole in the woman's skull, pushed up the temporal lobe – blood everywhere, gauze packed into the middle fossa, the ganglion cut, the wound closed and he was out of the house less than an hour after he had entered it.[11]

Readers would not have been surprised had Cushing concluded that Horsley was back home in time for lunch. But then others who worked with England's premier neurosurgeon remarked that neither surgical precision nor courteousness was sacrificed for speed. A junior member of his team, Ernest Jones, wrote that ward visits with the professor 'were accomplished in half the usual time but [Horsley] gave [each patient] the impression that he was his sole care in life and he would arrange their pillows with a tender deftness'.[12]

James B must have been sufficiently pleased with the plumpness of his pillows and Horsley's bedside manner to accompany the surgeon that summer (along with two other patients he'd similarly operated on) to attend a huge conference of the BMA in the Royal Pavilion at Brighton, the former summer palace of George IV. More than a thousand medical men from around the globe, including Charcot, descended on the south coast of England, drawn especially by tales of Horsley's success. In a pageant of pathology, James B and the other patients were put on public display; their case histories were presented in unsparing detail, and photographic illustrations of each stage of the operations were shown by lantern.

Horsley's presentation electrified the audience. The event came to be celebrated as a landmark in medical history. A decade after John Eric Erichsen had counselled that surgeons were in danger of over-reaching themselves, the same Erichsen now sat amongst the audience in Brighton and marvelled at Horsley's achievement as 'the most remarkable application of pure science to practical surgery that has ever been brought to the notice of the profession, one that opens a new era, that of cerebral surgery'.[13]

Horsley took to the Brighton seafront to walk off the heady excitement, his ears still ringing from the adulation of his peers, and to 'allow the boiling in his brain, aroused by the enthusiastic reception of his paper, to settle down'.[14] Few would have begrudged him his moment of cheer, and the chance temporarily to step out of character. After all, a doctor's register of emotions is mostly calibrated so that he remains sanguine, especially when dealing with patients when things go wrong. For, if there is no pity in medicine, much of the landscape *is* pitiful. And as Horsley was to discover, if he didn't already know, each surgeon carries a mental ledger that includes significant failures marked up alongside the triumphs.

Neurosurgery was still in its infancy as the nineteenth century crossed into the twentieth. Only a handful of surgeons were willing or able to conduct such delicate and complicated operations on the brain, and this was to create a dilemma for Horsley. A few years later, when attending a concert at the Royal Albert Hall, Horsley's adolescent son, Siward, collapsed and convulsed. A diagnosis of epilepsy was made. There were further fits on the following days. The records do not reveal the extent of his epilepsy or the violence of the fits but surgery was advised; and it fell to Horsley himself to undertake the onerous operation on his son. The procedure was successful. But Siward was not as lucky as James B. The fits abated, only to return within the year.

There was much sympathy for the invidious position Horsley found himself in as father and surgeon: 'How could he have borne to be visited, through his own son,' speculated David Taylor, 'with what he had laboured so fiercely to conquer in his patients?'[15]

Surgeons then as now walk a fine line between hubris and the demands on their skill stretched beyond the limits of what is possible. As René Leriche was to observe, 'Every surgeon carries about him a little cemetery, in which from time to time he goes to pray, a cemetery of bitterness and regret, in which he seeks the reason for certain of his failures.'[16] But surely, even if Siward was a good candidate for surgery, the reasons for Horsley's failure to cure his son were a consequence of the imprecision of neurosurgery at that time. Neurologists could at least be specific in language. New words and phrases emerged to help make sense of what they were seeing: 'aphasia', 'hysteroid', 'dreamy state' – both clumsy and elegant, the words became part of a new lexicon that is still in common usage. Nineteenth-century case notes from the National Hospital strikingly reveal the same language and attention to detail that is shown by physicians today.

It was such attention to history-taking that enabled doctors to begin to distinguish between epileptic fits and 'hysterical' seizures brought about through psychological disturbance in the patient. Though, given the standard treatments on offer – bromides for epileptic seizures versus metallic clamps around the groin for the falling women – the so-called hysteric might have benefited from being misdiagnosed with epilepsy. Further detachment from the then still-common perception which equated epilepsy with madness came also when people with epilepsy stopped being consigned to lunatic asylums.

More generally, the great breakthrough in understanding the range and nuances of epilepsy came about simply because, as inpatients, people with epilepsy could be closely monitored in ways that had never been possible or considered before. For the first time in medicine seizures were systematically described by nurses and doctors – one of them even gave his name to a type of seizure (Jacksonian) he'd best described. In Jacksonian seizures the tremors began in a patient's hands and 'marched' up her arms and body to her head. Jackson traced the tremors to lesions of the motor region of the cerebral cortex.

If the senior staff at the National Hospital knew themselves to be pioneers, then Jackson was first among equals. It is said that his interest in neurology began when he awoke one morning to discover that one side of his face was paralysed: he was suffering from Bell's palsy.[7] His interest began with himself and continued thereafter. Wherever he went, Jackson's curiosity preceded him. 'He stood with his head to the side,' wrote Macdonald Critchley, 'like a giant quizzical bird.'[18]

On the few unfortunate occasions that I was summoned to the dean's office, I had time to study, on the interminably long walk down the dimly lit corridor, the frieze of black-and-white photos that decorated the walls. Stiff-collared, earnest physicians looked down in judgement, it seemed; one walked a gauntlet of their gravitas. Each trepidatious step from one portrait to the next was a preparation for the solemn audience with the dean and a reminder of the high-minded ideals of one's chosen profession. Or so I thought. I didn't then know about the Bell's palsy which would have compromised or limited Hughling Jackson's expressions on one side. I didn't see in his face in the photo then what I see now: kindness, reserve but also a little mischief.

A 1904 group portrait at Queen Square shows two dozen or so physicians arranged in rows and in order of seniority, erect in their unyielding Victorian suits. All is as you might expect, perhaps. But on close inspection the appearance of one of the men belies the formality of the setting. Sitting in the front row, Hughlings Jackson's legs stick out, carefree, crossed at the feet. A few other biographical clues about the bushy-bearded neurologist hint at eccentricity. He's a fidgety man who tears off the hardback covers from books because he's only interested in the information, the content within; he rarely completes a full journey by train, but breaks off midway to change to a horse and carriage; and he never sits through both halves of a play, but leaves after the first half to return to the theatre on another day for the second. Finally he is cast as the archetypical absent-minded boffin who horrifies the dinner party when he pulls a handkerchief from his breast pocket and a piece of brain tissue drops onto the table. None of the stories detract from the appreciation of Jackson's skills as a physician; rather they're told with the fond regard that the English reserve for the eccentric.

There are myriad references to Jackson's elusive character and to suggestions that he was happier to be at the margins than centre stage. Awestruck contemporaries, who witnessed the first operation on a patient with epilepsy (James B), describe Horsley at the operating theatre: tense, erect, ready to pounce as soon as the patient has surrendered to the anaesthetising effect of the ether; whilst Hughlings Jackson looks on beneficently from the wings.

Medics' proximity to patients and ill health can give them a peculiar perspective on life. When you are routinely made aware of all that can go wrong with your body, you begin to see the threat of pathology everywhere; amongst my fellow medical students it induced a kind of paranoia. You learnt about a condition one week and believed you were succumbing to it yourself the following week. Throughout your time in medicine that knowledge, like a flint of disappointment, lingers in the corner of your mind's eye, and though saddened you are not surprised when tragedy eventually does strike.

The fate of Siward Horsley understandably cast a pall over his father's life. But amongst staff at the National Hospital there were several other incidents involving people with epilepsy when protocol and decorum were strained and the distance between patients and doctors collapsed. In his initial research into epilepsy Jackson identified two basic types of seizure: focal motor (where there was an obvious start to the fits in some distant part of the body); and psychomotor seizures (associated with déjà vu which Jackson termed the 'dreamy state').

The first paper of Jackson's in the journal *Brain* on this latter class of dreamy-state seizures centred on a patient who unusually had written and published, under the pseudonym Quaerens (seeker), an account of his own epileptic experiences. As well as being a neighbour of Jackson's, the seeker was also a fellow physician. The twenty-six-year-old Quaerens presented himself to Jackson in 1877. For a neurologist grappling with the enigma of epilepsy, who hoped to collate individual stories to establish patterns so that the specific might eventually yield collective insights into the universal characteristics of the condition, Quaerens offered an exciting and unprecedented case study. Jackson discreetly referred to him subsequently as 'Dr Z' in a number of academic papers in which he transcribed how his patient's epilepsy had evolved.[19]

At first Dr Z, a young energetic sportsman of vim and vigour (cricketer, tennis player and climber) paid little attention to his increasing propensity to be subjected to a number of uncanny and unbidden thoughts. If anything he was amused by these instances of minor mental interference 'regarding the matter playfully as of no practical importance'. On one occasion at university when idly waiting for a friend he wrote, 'My attention was suddenly absorbed in my own mental state, of a vivid and unexpected recollection – of what I do not know'; on another he found himself reading a poem and anticipating the next line 'verbatim' even though he'd never read the poem before.

Jackson was impressed by the keenness of his patient's intellect; by his ability, for instance, to connect his own experiences to the common perception of déjà vu as articulated by Charles Dickens. 'We have all some experience of a feeling which comes over us occasionally,' wrote Dickens in *David Copperfield*, 'of our knowing perfectly what will be said next, as if we suddenly remembered it.' On its own déjà vu would not be a signifier of epilepsy but along with absences and unconscious automatic action it most certainly was. Indeed, Dr Z was more disturbed by the odd moments of lost time when he'd obviously carried out some activity that he couldn't subsequently account for.

In a game of tennis, for instance, though his opponent had not noticed any drop-off in his ability to continue a rally, Dr Z later confessed he'd had no memory of playing any strokes for the last few minutes. Then there was the time when as a young doctor he paid a home visit to a sickly child, took out his stethoscope for the examination, and then found himself at a table in the next room writing out a prescription, yet had no recollection of having made a diagnosis. But even that episode paled beside his dramatic account of running across a Swiss glacier in 1878 when he felt a seizure coming on and was unable to stop, yet felt 'no fear, but only a slight interest in what would happen'. He endured the queer sensations of petit mal, regained his composure and was surprised when looking back to see that he had run over the long slope of broken ice without injury, 'picking my way, I know not how, over ground that would normally have been difficult to me'.

Dr Z, who a century later was identified as Arthur T. Myers, was a star in the firmament of nineteenth-century medical case histories. His condition – common knowledge in the profession – was kept from the public. Myers's own inquisitiveness into the characteristics of his epilepsy was as piqued as Jackson's. But his reflections on the theory of the unconscious also led him into more fanciful territory, writing critically for the newly found Society for Psychical Research on matters related to the psychic or paranormal.[20]

As a young man Dr Z had engendered great expectations that he would excel in his profession, but epilepsy was an impediment to his medical ambitions. He'd hoped but failed to gain an appointment at a teaching hospital; and as his epilepsy worsened so his reliance on the sedative chloral hydrate increased.

A decade after being taken on as a patient by Jackson, Arthur T. Myers died from an excessive intake of chloral hydrate. A number of scholars have advanced the view that Myers committed suicide by taking an overdose of the drug. There was no hint of it in the *BMJ*'s obituary but then that journal was even coy about his epilepsy. Mourning his loss, the obituarist wrote, 'Destiny thought fit to inflict upon him that terrible and inscrutable nervous malady which occasionally harassed him in early youth, and of late years advanced with relentless tread, baffling the most devoted medical skill, and ultimately involving a fine intellect in ruin and confusion.'[21]

Myers's apparent suicide exercised Hughlings Jackson, not only because of the tragedy of a patient taking his own life but because Myers's death and subsequent autopsy carried with them the potential to yield a secret; for Jackson to explore his suspicions about the site/seat in the brain of his patient's epilepsy. For as well as the déjà vu and absences, Dr Z had demonstrated peculiar yet subtle lip-smacking and other gestures that Jackson associated with his epilepsy. And in animal experiments David Ferrier (Jackson's colleague) had shown how these actions corresponded to certain discrete parts of the brain.

A decade after Jackson had first set eyes on Myers he now attended his autopsy, and fired by the opportunity and risk it presented 'begged [the pathologist] Dr. Colman to search the taste region of Ferrier on each half of the brain very carefully'. And lo and behold, 'Dr. Colman found a very small focus of softening in that region (in the uncinate gyrus) of the left half of the brain.' With the posthumous help of Dr Z, his physician John Hughlings Jackson had made a remarkable discovery which was hugely to advance the understanding of epilepsy: the peculiar lip-smacking 'movements of the mouth and tongue' witnessed in Dr Z's seizures were the 'indirect "reflex" results of an epileptic discharge beginning in gustatory elements of a certain region of the brain – the taste region of Ferrier', in the temporal lobes of the cerebral cortex. Today it is known as temporal lobe epilepsy.[22]

John Hughlings Jackson was a generous man. His reticence in naming Arthur Myers owed much not just to doctor–patient confidentiality but also to the kind of reserve typical of the Victorian age. Had Jackson been working today and attending to Myers he would have celebrated an unspoken collaboration in the manner of Oliver Sacks acknowledging the importance to medicine of the man who mistook his wife for a hat.

But what is also extraordinary about John Hughlings Jackson's neurological findings is that he *was* working in the dark; without the benefit of EEG (still many decades away from development); with no means of attaching electrodes to the scalp or implanting intracranial electrodes on the brain to allow for precise neuro imaging; but simply through close observation and a process of deduction, Hughlings Jackson divined the basic brain mechanisms through which seizures occurred. His description of a seizure as 'an occasional sudden excessive, rapid and local discharge in the grey matter [of the brain]' became the standard. Its simplicity is striking but there were several iterations and much refining before Hughlings Jackson was satisfied with the truth and elegance of that sentence.

Hughlings Jackson realised, as do we now, that though his focus was epilepsy, the larger purpose of his research was the workings of the brain:

> He who is faithfully analysing many different cases of epilepsy is doing far more than studying epilepsy. The highest centres ('organ of mind'), those concerned in such fits, represent all, literally all, parts of the body sensorially and motorially, in most complex ways, in most intricate combinations, etc. A careful study of many varieties of epileptic fits is one way of analysing this kind of representation by the 'organ of mind'.[23]

He sought a grand theory to explain brain function. To do so he looked to Charles Darwin and more importantly to Herbert Spencer, the philosopher who had influenced Darwin and had coined the term the 'survival of the fittest'.

Jackson borrowed from evolutionary theory to postulate his own theory of the hierarchy of the brain; he suggested that there were higher levels of the brain that restrained the lower levels. If those restrictions were lifted then that might lead to the expression of disease, in the same way that governments imposed order on nations and if their governance was breached disorder would ensue.

To some the qualifications and sub-clauses in Jackson's writing served only to make the essays and papers obscure. His unwieldy penmanship was likened by a friend to a barely controlled team of horses threatening constantly to shoot off in different directions. But it is always easier to say what something is not rather than to say what something is – to bring into the culture an idea or expression that has not surfaced before. Jackson's style was clear enough; and where inspiration failed him he borrowed and acknowledged the debt. For example, in their essays, a number of nineteenth-century neurologists, Jackson included, explored the latency of seizures by using the metaphor of the unexploded potential of gunpowder. There was synchronicity, too, with great authors such as Dostoevsky in his depiction of epilepsy in fiction. The language of Dostoevsky and Hughlings Jackson was uncannily similar. Both men were able to conjure for readers the spooky 'dreamy states' and 'forced thinking' of epilepsy.

During consultations Hughlings Jackson had a reputation for bluntness or at any rate of deliberately not adding a sugar coating to any prognosis. There were also tales of him hurrying past the beds of patients whom he thought he could not help. But if, in addressing patients, he seemed guilty of overt dispassion, it was not from a lack of empathy towards them; he just sought precision and clarity in language; a spade by any other name was still a spade.

As a medical student I was often struck by the coded language used in hospitals that had at times a waggish schoolboy quality. A contemporary of Jackson, a neurologist called Radcliffe, famously described a patient having a seizure as 'being strangled by the bow [string] of an invisible executioner'. Notwithstanding its dramatic impact, the language suggests a hangover of the dark humour cultivated by some in medicine. Jackson, though an intellectual, was more inclined towards plain language.

On 25 July 1865, John Hughlings Jackson plainly declared his love and devotion to his first cousin Elizabeth Dade Jackson (a children's author) by marrying her. A decade into their marriage, Elizabeth died at the age of thirty-nine, following childbirth in which her baby also died. An editorial in the journal *Brain* revealed that 'Jackson observed the type of seizure named after him in his own wife who developed a cerebral sinus thrombosis during her puerperium from which she perished.'[24] That short sentence carries the intriguing suggestion that one of the people from whom John Hughlings Jackson gleaned his masterful observations of epilepsy was his wife. Jackson's diaries and casebooks might have confirmed this but such correspondence was never archived. After Elizabeth's death, her husband was even less inclined to socialise. A place was always kept for Elizabeth at the dining table on the rare occasions when visitors called. He never remarried. From 1876 onwards medicine was his wife.

Jackson never wrote a book (he didn't have the kind of temperament required for such sustained endeavour on a single subject). But he was prolific in his writing output, contributing several hundred essays and papers to journals such as *Brain* and the *BMJ*. For more than a decade the pages of the *Lancet* were graced by a series of Jackson's disconnected notes, 'Neurological Fragments', that were largely ruminations on any subject that took his fancy, from intracranial syphilis to the psychology of joking. For such a prodigious writer, Jackson's last will and testament was very odd and intriguing. He left instructions to 'destroy all my letters and diaries and all my case books and all correspondence relating thereto'.

John Hughlings Jackson was never knighted for services to medicine as were a number of his peers. But his profession held him in the highest regard – in England and beyond. The term 'Jacksonian seizure' entered the medical lexicon largely because of the advocacy of his contemporary, Jean-Martin Charcot. The French neurologist was also central to this phase of the story of epilepsy, in particular in his efforts to determine the boundaries of the condition; to draw a distinction, for instance, between organic seizures resulting from epilepsy and hysterical seizures resulting from psychological disturbances.

From the early 1860s Charcot presided over the neuropsychiatric hospital, La Salpêtrière, an institution that was largely a repository for hysterics, epileptics, and the insane, all lumped together without formal differential diagnosis. There Charcot gained an international reputation alongside Hughlings Jackson's. Charcot's fame grew out of his public lectures and demonstrations of hypnotised hysterics. The masterclasses were hugely popular and drew audiences from around Europe, among them a young Dr Sigmund Freud from Vienna.

Up until Charcot there had been an unresolved confusion of the nature (if at all) of the relationship between epilepsy and hysteria. Charcot claimed through careful observation to have isolated and identified hysteria as a distinct entity separate from epilepsy; as well as discovering a new disorder which he called 'hystero-epilepsy' (incorporating epileptic aspects into the crisis of hysteria). The symptoms included 'convulsions, contortions, fainting, and transient impairment of consciousness', which Charcot demonstrated to his medical students on ward rounds at La Salpêtrière.

Charcot became obsessed with hysteria. In his estimation far greater numbers of his patients suffered from hysteria than from epilepsy. Only later would Charcot's diagnoses be more sharply criticised as the function of the 'practitioners' preferences' – a thinly veiled code for blinkered bias.

It would fall to a sceptical student to convince Charcot that he had invented rather than discovered hystero-epilepsy; that the signs, symptoms and behaviour exhibited by the patients at La Salpêtrière came about from the persuasive power of suggestion from Charcot and his luminaries.

The confusion over hysteria and epilepsy was eventually cleared up, but over the next century the doubts over the boundaries between epilepsy and mental ill health remained. Even today within the medical profession, there are a number of neurologists who, though content to treat epilepsy, are anxious to ring-fence their discipline to prevent the leakage of psychiatric complaints. All of which occasionally leads to suspected epileptics shuffling between the two camps. And further complications arise when people with epilepsy, such as Christopher, struggling to come to terms with their condition, either solicit help or behave in ways which lead to involuntary medical interventions.

The phone rang again. It was just after midnight. I knew even before picking up the receiver that the call would be related to Christopher. This time it was a ward sister from St Clement's Hospital. I knew St Clement's. I'd spent a few months as a student working on its acute wards. It was an old psychiatric hospital (and former workhouse) that fell under the remit of the London. I couldn't fully hold on to what the ward sister was saying. I was distracted by her warm syrupy West Indian accent, and by the unnerving conviction that I knew her; and that perhaps she knew me.

Sometimes when you bump into an acquaintance outside their normal environment, both people immediately and unilaterally arrive at the decision that the best course of action is to pretend not to recognise each other. Having made such a decision it is impossible to go back. This seemed such a moment.

The ward sister did not acknowledge that she knew me but her tone suggested the opposite: she was gentle and sympathetic.

'Colin – I can call you Colin?'

'Yes.'

'Your brother need some help, Colin.'

I had the impression that she was speaking in code.

'You think him need some help?' she asked.

'Help?'

'Yes, Colin. You can help him. It's not too late. If you come now. It must be now. If it was later, Colin. Well, it might be too late. Y'understan'?'

'What's he saying?'

'Hmmm. Well, him not all that talkative. He just say he surrender.'

'Surrenders?'

'Mmm hmm. So, you coming? Or you rather we keep him?'

I balanced the receiver between my ear and shoulder and pulled an arm through the sleeve of my jacket. I didn't answer the sister but tried instead to push away an ugly thought that had entered my mind when considering her question, 'Or you rather we keep him?'

Ticket to Heaven

The man stood out because he was white; the congregation was black. No one could recall him coming into the hall, but, odder still, later no one remembered him leaving. Dale Road in Luton was not known as a place where the devil would have the gall to reveal himself. For Dale Road (as we called it) was a Pentecostal church, frequented by my mother and siblings. Satan would not find recruits amongst the believers there but it didn't stop him trying; as my mother used to say, 'The devil is a bad man.'

Occasionally, when home, I was roped into picking up the family after service. On this occasion I arrived late into a melee of churchgoers in the midst of some commotion. A man I feared was Christopher but could not get close enough to be sure, writhed on the floor in front of the stage, in the throes of a grand mal seizure. People backed away from him, panicking and in horror; until fearless church elders closed in on the man. All believed that evil had entered his body and taken over the poor wretch; and the jerks and spasms marked his futile attempts to wrestle with this alien invasion.

At the height of the commotion people began whispering about the white stranger in a dark suit who'd entered the building and had sat by himself at the back of the church, separated from the congregation by four or five empty rows. He had disappeared but his dark work was now made manifest.

The regular pastor was on holiday and his replacement had no experience of exorcism. He instructed two of the elders to lift up the fallen brother, to stretch his arms around their necks and to walk with him, as if he were a drunken reveller who could be sobered up by walking it off. It was Christopher, as I suspected. I couldn't move, but it wasn't just the swell of people that stopped me from getting close to him; the drama repelled me. I was loath to enter into it, and tried vainly to push aside thoughts of denial and betrayal, of Peter and Christ and a cock crowing. Christopher, I reasoned, would forgive me. It would be over soon enough.

All the while the congregation was weeping and wailing whilst the two elders called upon God to free Christopher from the devil's grip. It was 1989 in my brother's nineteenth year; and I could not save him from the church's intervention.

The relationship between religion and epilepsy has not been a happy one. For much of human history, God-fearing populations have associated epilepsy negatively with demonic possession. Rather than being pitied, people with epilepsy inspired terror.

The longevity of that prevailing attitude, as exemplified by the elders of Dale Road, has its roots in a biblical story, in the Gospel according to Mark. A man appeals to Jesus for help with his son who 'hath a dumb spirit; and wheresoever he taketh him, he teareth him; and he foameth and gnasheth with his teeth and pineth away . . .' Jesus demands to see the boy and immediately the man's son collapses into some kind of seizure. Jesus then questions the father some more and learns about the boy's history of paroxysms that have led dangerously at times to him falling into fires or water. It's clearly a difficult case. 'This kind of demon is not cast out but by prayer and fasting,' says Jesus. And only once he has established that the father is a believer does he rebuke 'the foul, unclean spirits', and charge them to 'come out of him and enter no more'. The boy emits an epileptic cry and drops down as if dead. But, records Mark, 'Jesus took him by the hand, and lifted him up; and he arose.'[1]

The boy, whose epilepsy is never mentioned, is cleansed and resurrected to a state of grace. The unclean spirits were proxy for the devil. People with epilepsy were both unclean and contagious. Only a fool would go near them. 'We are in the habit of spitting as a preservative from epilepsy,' wrote the Roman scholar Pliny, 'and we repel contagion thereby.'[2] More generally, the sight of someone having a fit was taken as a bad omen. Amongst the Romans, as previously noted, it was cause enough for the cancellation of public meetings. But even so, the notion of equating epilepsy with demonic possession is relatively modern. Ancient Greece did not cast such aspersions on people who fell down and convulsed but only held that they were obviously cursed by one of the gods who, in his wrath at some transgression, had visited them with an incurable 'Sacred Disease'. Getting on the wrong side of Selene, the goddess of the moon, for example, would mark you down for epilepsy. The association of the moon with the condition continued throughout ancient history till medieval times. And in antiquity, if you didn't know which Greek god you'd offended then your subsequent symptoms would give you a clue. If the patient's epileptic cry resembled a horse's scream, for example, it suggested Poseidon was the offended party.[3]

One of the first mentions of the 'Sacred Disease' in literature appears in the writing of the historian Herodotus. In the *Histories*, Herodotus tries to clear up the myth behind the illness of the Persian King Cambyses II who was said to have been smitten with insanity/epilepsy in divine retribution for his sacrilegious killing of the Egyptian bull-deity, Apis. Writing almost a century after the death of Cambyses, Herodotus distances himself from the popular conception of a sacred disease: 'Thus was Cambyses mad against his own kindred, whether because of the Apis bull, or because of some other of the many calamities which tend to fall upon men; for they say that Cambyses suffered by heredity from a terrible disease which some call "sacred"; for it is not likely that the mind should remain healthy when the body is suffering from a great illness.'[4]

At no time does Herodotus question the popular association of epilepsy with mental ill health, but when it comes to a religious connection he hedges his bets with the qualification 'some call sacred'. Herodotus was aware that Greek physicians from as early as 400 BC were sceptical about the superstitious link between epilepsy and religion. The collection of anonymous physicians who wrote under the name Hippocrates stated bluntly that epilepsy was no more sacred than any other disease. In the Hippocratic text *On Sacred Disease* – an attack on the conjurors, charlatans and mountebanks who shelter behind ignorance to peddle their magical potions – the author wrote, 'Men regard [epilepsy's] nature and cause as divine from ignorance and wonder, because it is not at all like other diseases. And this notion of its divinity is kept up by their inability to comprehend it, and the simplicity of the mode by which it is cured, for men are freed from it by purifications and incantations.'[5]

Some scholars believe that epilepsy's description as a sacred disease also has its roots in the tragedy of the divine Heracles. One tradition holds that Heracles' epileptic affliction was brought on by his prodigious labours. In an account attributed to Aristotle, black bile (associated with epilepsy) is said to have caused the mental derangement in Heracles that led to him killing his wife and children.[6]

Over time spitting out/at the contagion of the unclean spirits would not be enough, as people with epilepsy came to be seen not just as a passive vessel for the demons but also active agents for evil. Why run the risk of not being able to exorcise the demons? It was safer to kill the proxy.

During the Middle Ages, people with epilepsy were rounded up in the hunt for witches. The *Malleus Maleficarum*, the popular manual for witch-hunters and Inquisitors, published initially by a pair of Dominican monks in 1487, argued that 'there is no bodily infirmity, not even leprosy or epilepsy, which cannot be caused by witches, with God's permission'.[7] Any inexplicable malady then could be, and often was, attributed to magic; and witches, the handmaidens of this magic, might visit on the unfortunate victims the very condition that they perhaps suffered from themselves. If both witch and the possessed demonstrated similar signs and symptoms (of epilepsy) then how could they be distinguished? Often they could not. And indeed one of the common characteristics of witches, according to the *Malleus Maleficarum*, was a propensity towards seizures. The wisdom of such an assertion was not up for debate (doubters were obviously in the service of the devil). If there were myriad examples to choose from to illustrate the point, so too were the means of transmission many – potions, spells, even eggs. 'For we have often found that certain people have been visited with epilepsy or the falling sickness by means of eggs which have been buried with dead bodies, especially the dead bodies of witches.'

No doubt there were instances of settling of scores; of people with epilepsy being denounced because their grand mal seizures offended the sensibilities of the burghers of their town; others confessed, even before setting eyes on the rack, that they were in league with the devil: of course they were guilty; they must have brought the diabolic seizures on themselves; why else would they have been forsaken by the Lord? The appetite for righteous persecution did not wane for several hundred years during which thousands of people were executed.

The zealous pursuit of witches and warlocks and the clash between epilepsy and religion was not confined to the West. Abu al-Qasim Khalaf ibn 'Abbas az-Zahrawi, one of the most famous surgeons of the medieval Islamic world, listed five causes of epilepsy. The fifth culprit was 'some outside agent whose mode [of action] is not known, and is said to be caused, as usual, by *allahin ablis* (demons).[8]

Possession could take hold of both the sinner and the saint; the agents of the devil and the emissaries of God. The distinction was not always so clearly drawn between the two: between those cursed with evil spirits and visionaries invested with supernatural powers to do God's bidding on earth. Both, in their uncanny behaviour and eerie spasmodic gestures, demonstrated possession.

A sixteenth-century scholar, Méric Casaubon, recorded several accounts of people whose epilepsy allegedly endowed them with prophetic powers. One of the most memorable was an apprentice baker who, having been beaten brutally by his master, was left with a head injury that resulted in a succession of epileptic seizures. The fits gave way to ecstasies in which he later claimed to have seen dead relatives in paradise. Once the fits had abated, 'when he was perfectly come to himself . . . then would he sadly and with much confidence maintain that he had been not upon his bed, as they that were present would make him believe; but in heaven with his Heavenly Father . . . When he foresaw his fits coming upon him, he would say that now the Angels were ready to carry him away.'[9]

When the apprentice was later denounced as a fraud, he might well have pleaded that such was the prophet's lot. It was certainly the case for one of his predecessors, a nineteen-year-old French peasant who, after proclaiming visions and insisting that she was instructed with messages from God, was burned at the stake in

1432, following her trial for heresy. It was beyond dispute that angels (as she alleged) could communicate with people, but were the voices she heard from God or the devil? Two years earlier, Joan of Arc, the peasant girl, now clad in special armour, had led a French army that managed miraculously in four days to lift the siege of Orléans. But when she attempted the same again at Compiègne several months later, she was captured by the Burgundians and their English allies and put on trial. The enemy sought to discredit the woman they called the 'Armagnac whore', a heretic who had deviated from the Church's doctrine. Her interrogation, then, turned on theology. The devil might be spied in the detail of her testimony, with her prosecutors focusing on the nature of the spirits to challenge the authenticity of her visions.

At no time during her trial was it suggested that Joan of Arc might have been suffering from epilepsy but, though far from unanimous, that is the belief of a number of contemporary neurological experts. To their colleagues in psychiatry, Joan of Arc's visions might best be explained as the kind of command hallucinations familiar in psychosis; but neurologists, such as Elizabeth Foote-Smith and Lydia Bayne, have made a compelling case that her visions were examples of epileptic ecstatic auras. The clues, they say, are in Joan of Arc's court testimony of her visions, in which the sound of church bells precedes the Voice of God. The first time that Joan heard the voice she was fearful:

It was mid-day, in the summer, in my father's garden . . . I heard this voice to my right, towards the Church, rarely do I hear it, without its being accompanied also by a light. The light comes from the same side as the Voice. Generally, it is a great light . . . When I heard it for the third time, I recognised that it was the Voice of an Angel. This voice always guarded me well, and I have always understood it; it instructed me to be good and to go often to Church; it told me it was necessary for me to come into France . . . it said to me two or three times a week: 'You must go into France.' . . . It said to me: 'Go, raise the siege which is being made before the City of Orléans. Go!' . . . and I replied that I was but a poor girl, who knew nothing of riding and fighting . . . There is never a day when I do not hear this Voice; and I have much need of it.

The neurologists believe that Joan of Arc's account of the ringing church bells which preceded her visions is redolent of musicogenic epilepsy in which music is the stimulus that provokes seizures. In Joan's case the fact that she also reported visions (hallucinations) without any physical component (i.e. convulsions) suggests temporal lobe epilepsy. Other features also point to epilepsy – the discrete episodic nature of the visual hallucinations, though frightening to her at first, were ultimately ecstatic and subsequently welcomed by her. Indeed, she regretted their passing.

Over the centuries, researchers have advanced a range of other medical conditions as the possible root cause of Joan of Arc's visions. But whilst any retrospective diagnosis can only be speculative, Foote-Smith and Bayne strengthen their case by ruling out candidates such as migraine and psychosis, and instead flagging up, for example, Joan's elation and grandiosity (which sustained her throughout the seven years from her first recorded vision to her execution), as well as her diminished or hypo-sexuality as further associated signs and symptoms to underscore a possible diagnosis of epilepsy.

At the end of her trial, taken to the square in Rouen to be executed, Joan of Arc suddenly recanted; she submitted to the authorities and was returned to her cell (to begin a life sentence).

But days later she withdrew her confession. She would not, she said, damn her soul to save her life. Joan could not and would not deny her voices and apparitions and the meaning that she attached to them. She was taken back to the execution square, tied to a stake and burned at the pyre on 30 May 1431.

The court had challenged the veracity of her visions theologically. Accepted doctrine held that visions of angels could only be spiritual, yet Joan was adamant that the angels that had visited her were corporeal, were as real in body as any human. Ultimately the hallucinations had been so powerful and so vivid that they had fuelled her convictions.

Neurologists argue that there are numerous instances in history, contemporaneously and for years later described as revelations or visions, for which our modern understanding of epilepsy and the workings of the brain now offers the chance to make a retrospective diagnosis. God-fearing believers cry that this sort of rethinking detracts from the poignancy of such tales and the remarkable events that followed such visions. They cite the case of Saul of Tarsus whose inspiring legacy of the power of religious conversion, as illustrated by his visions, is threatened by the prosaic interpretation of epileptic hallucinations.

Saul was a Pharisee, a zealous Jew, renowned for his unstinting pursuit and prosecution of the early followers of Jesus. In AD 34 he took to the road, on a journey to Damascus, in the year following Christ's crucifixion, to apprehend members of this new Messianic sect and to bring them to trial in Jerusalem. But as he neared the city 'suddenly a light from heaven flashed around him'. He fell to the ground and heard a voice say to him, 'Saul, Saul, why do you persecute me?'

'Who are you, Lord?' Saul asked.

'I am Jesus, whom you are persecuting,' he replied. 'Now get up and go into the city, and you will be told what you must do.'

Two thousand years after the event it is perhaps stretching credibility to take an enigmatic account of a solitary episode of audiovisual hallucination (blinding light coupled with the voice of Jesus) as evidence of epilepsy, but neurologists who do so also enlist the story of Saul's other visons and ecstatic auras to support their case.

In a letter to the Church in Corinth, Saul (now Paul the Apostle) recounts further ecstatic experiences when he was 'caught up to the third heaven. In the body or out of the body? That I do not know . . . I simply know that . . . [I]was caught up to paradise and heard sacred secrets which no human lips can repeat. Of an experience like that I am prepared to boast . . . My wealth of visions might have puffed me up, so I was given a thorn in the flesh, an angel of Satan to rack me and keep me from being puffed up.'

Unpacking this account from a medical perspective, some neurologists conclude that Paul is describing other psychic and perceptual experiences of temporal lobe epilepsy; the ecstasy of otherworldly (in/out of body) auras is tempered later by the agony (thorn in the flesh) of subsequent convulsive seizures.

Science is often accused of a cold revisionism. Keats famously complained that Newton had spoiled the poetry of the rainbow by reducing it to the prismatic colours. But is a rational, scientific explanation of an epileptic attack for Saul's Damascene conversion any less a thing of beauty and wonder than the biblical tale?

Theologians, such as the Bishop of Durham, argue against the 'reductionist way of explaining' profound expressions of spirituality. For followers and believers (my mother and siblings among them), exceptional figures such as Joan of Arc and Saul, after his conversion to Paul, acted as conduits for the Lord Almighty. God also spoke to the Black Moses, Harriet Tubman, and inspired her quest to liberate hundreds of her enslaved compadres at the height of the Atlantic slave trade. But were the prophets visionary or delusionary? Were they blessed, as few are, with hyper-religiosity or were they suffering from an illness, temporal lobe epilepsy perhaps, for which there was no diagnosis at that time, nor effective treatment?

Ecstatic hallucinations are rare. But similar-sounding accounts were given to the early nineteenth-century neurologists Gowers and Hughlings Jackson by patients who, prior to the attacks, professed to have no religious conviction. As is often the case in medicine, it was these more complex cases that intrigued neurologists. In his close study of epilepsy, and in particular when categorising auras, Hughlings Jackson drew a distinction between crude sensations (such as smell, sound and taste) and more sophisticated reminiscences or dreamy states. Patients struggled to describe the peculiar thoughts that arrived unbidden in these latter hallucinations which Hughlings Jackson considered to be elaborate and voluminous mental states. One patient, a twenty-nine-year-old man, was perplexed and disturbed by the curious sensation of his auras which were 'a sort of transplantation to another world, lasting a second or so'.

In the dreamy state, the patients did not necessarily lose consciousness; they suffered a defect of consciousness. But whereas the cruder seizures left patients in a negative mental state, here they were propelled into a super-positive state of increased, double or over-consciousness. And Jackson noted tellingly that the seizures were not always disagreeable; sometimes they were just the opposite: 'I have had patients say that they used to encourage the feeling before they knew what it meant.'

But what did it mean? Unlike the association of crude auras with specific parts of the brain, the neurologists could, at this stage, only theorise as to the location that gave rise to these spooky sensations. Matters were further complicated when the hallucinations were complex and neither finite nor discrete – as was the case for an intelligent young man who presented himself to Gowers with myriad sensations. Gowers recorded the patient's case history in his book *Epilepsy*: 'First there was a sensation . . . like pain with a cramp . . . pass[ing] up the left side of the chest with a "thump, thump" . . . The sensations rose up to the left ear, and then was like the "hissing of a railway engine", . . . then he suddenly and invariably saw before him an old woman in a stiff brown dress who offered him something which had the smell of Tonquin beans."[10] Gowers postulated that the complex sequence of sensations described by the patient reflected contiguous excessive discharges coursing across his brain. The motor, auditory and olfactory components of the seizure could be traced to discharges in the relative parts of the brain associated with those sensations but the origin of psychic component (the vision of the old woman) was as yet beyond medical understanding. For now neurologists, such as Gowers and Hughlings Jackson, confined themselves to descriptions of patients who likened the dreamy state to a way of perceiving the world simultaneously with 'two minds' or 'double consciousness'. Hughlings Jackson, recognising that this voluminous mental state was often accompanied by an aura, drew on his theory of a hierarchy of the brain (with the higher centres controlling the lower) to propose that the dreamy state resulted from a 'loss of control; and possibly may depend on [a] rise in activity on the opposite cerebral hemisphere'.[11]

About 2,000 kilometres to the east of London's National Hospital where Hughlings Jackson and Gowers transcribed and attempted to interpret the peculiar reminiscences and voluminous thoughts of some of their more complex cases, Fyodor Mikhailovich Dostoevsky, was, at about the same time, employing similar language to describe his own and his fictional characters' uncanny experiences of epilepsy. In a diary entry for 7 September 1880,

Dostoevsky recorded his mental state during a seizure: 'This morning at 8.45, interruption of my thoughts, transported into other years, dreams, dreamy states, dreaminess.'

The dreamy state had its attractions. In his novel *The Idiot* Dostoevsky's protagonist Prince Myshkin's debilitating epileptic seizures are occasionally compensated for by a moment of lucidity that precedes an attack:

> He was thinking, incidentally, that there was a moment or two in his epileptic condition almost before the fit itself (if it occurred in waking hours) when suddenly amid the sadness, spiritual darkness and depression, his brain seemed to catch fire at brief moments . . . His sensation of being alive and his awareness increased tenfold at those moments which flashed by like lightning. His mind and heart were flooded by a dazzling light. All his agitation, doubts and worries, seemed composed in a twinkling, culminating in a great calm, full of understanding . . . but these moments, these glimmerings were still but a premonition of that final second (never more than a second) with which the seizure itself began. That second was, of course, unbearable.

Dostoevsky was determined to witness and to give testimony to that which was unbearable. In his writing he began to perceive the possibility that his illness, all illness, was potentially a vehicle for transcendence: 'As soon as he falls ill, as soon as the normal healthy state of the organism is disturbed, the possibility of another world begins to appear,' wrote the novelist, 'and as the illness increases, so do the contacts with the other world."[12]

The first intimations of that other-worldliness and his contact with it began whilst he was in exile in Siberia serving a prison sentence for sedition. He was lucky to be alive. Along with his colleagues, he'd been blindfolded, put in front of a firing squad and subjected to a mock execution. Some scholars even suggest that the trauma was enough to have triggered his first seizure. Then, one Easter night, during his exile, Dostoevsky was visited by an old friend to whom he confided that he'd experienced a prophetic vision during an epileptic aura:

> The air was filled with a big noise and I tried to move. I felt the heaven was going down upon the earth, and that it had engulfed me. I have really touched God. He came into me myself; yes, God exists, I cried, you all, healthy people, have no idea what joy that joy is which we epileptics experience the second before a seizure. Mahomet, in his Koran, said he had seen Paradise and had gone into it. All these stupid clever men are quite sure that he was a liar and a charlatan. But no, he did not lie, he really had been in Paradise during an attack of epilepsy; he was a victim of this disease as I am. I do not know whether this joy lasts for seconds or hours or months, but believe me, I would not exchange it for all the delights of this world.

In the last two decades of his life up until 1880, Dostoevsky recorded the details of his 102 seizures. He sought not only to codify them, but to draw out their spiritual dimension; to establish their meaning and divine purpose. But was Dostoevsky a reliable witness? For many years after his death, Sigmund Freud was considered the authority on Dostoevsky's condition. In Freud's analysis Dostoevsky's epilepsy should be placed in inverted commas. His seizures were, Freud suggested, merely hysterical ones first brought on by the trauma surrounding the death of Dostoevsky's father. Freud elaborated on his theory in the essay 'Dostoevsky and Parricide', published in 1928: 'Dostoevsky called himself an epileptic . . . it is highly probable that this so-called epilepsy was only a symptom of his neurosis and must accordingly be classified as hysteron-epilepsy – that is severe hysteria. The most probable assumption is that the attacks went back far into his childhood, that their place was taken to begin with by milder symptoms and that they did not assume an epileptic form until after the shattering experience of his eighteenth year – the murder of his father.'

Freud's assertion runs counter to Dostoevsky's own account as well as that of the friends and physicians who attended him. But even if Freud's analysis is discounted, confusion remains over the nature or type of epilepsy suffered by Dostoevsky. He seems to have had both generalised and partial seizures – a number of them accompanied by revelatory auras. But why do people such as Dostoevsky have ecstatic hallucinations? Why ecstatic rather than the more common sensory varieties? Are the auras generated from a particular location in the brain whose stimulation elicits a response of hyper-religiosity or spirituality? Or might it not simply be that such people with epilepsy already have a predisposition to hyper-religiosity? After all, Joan of Arc's piety preceded her visions (when she was working in the fields any sound of church bells would cause her to drop to her knees in prayer); Saul's visions occurred when he was already embarked on a spiritual journey that would test his faith and conviction.

As with all retrospective, historical diagnoses the evidence is soft. Today, in attempting to understand seizures (spiritual or otherwise), we are more inclined to look for clues in the laboratory than literature; to divine awe in the science rather than the poetry. Greater clarity would come half a century after Dostoevsky's death with the electroencephalogram, a tool that was introduced in 1929 for measuring changes in the electrical field on the scalp. Through electroencephalography, neurologists would gain much greater insights into the electrical activity deep within the brain during seizures.

It wasn't long before neurologists conceived that if probes could register neurological discharges in the brain, they might also be used to pass down harmless electrical currents to mimic those discharges.

In 1938 the neurologist Wilder Penfield conducted a series of experiments using probes to electrically stimulate the region of the temporal lobes (situated either side of the cerebrum, behind the temples) of patients with epilepsy. Inserting the probes under local anaesthesia, Penfield was able to reproduce in the patients past experiences that had occurred regularly as part of their dreamy-state seizure patterns – whether as reminiscences or déjà vu. More surprisingly, Penfield also noted that prior happenings unrelated to any previous epileptic attacks were also recalled when the surgical electrode was applied.[13] When the experiments were conducted again a decade later they achieved the same results; and in 1963 Penfield and his researchers were further able to delimit the area – that is, to get even closer to the location in the temporal lobe suspected to be responsible for the psychical hallucination of sound, vision, and familiarity – 'a sudden re-experiencing of the past', or, for example, 'a sudden false interpretation of the present'.

One of the researchers' goals was to advance the work of Hughlings Jackson, to begin to classify the varieties of hallucinations that he had termed dreamy states. They settled on three broad categories: automatism (amnesia, confusion), interpretive signal (illusion, déjà vu), and experiential hallucination (flashback). The 1963 study was part of a large-scale review of the records of over a thousand patients at the Montreal Neurological Institute who'd been operated on for the relief of partial (focal) epilepsy over the last thirty years. In particular it would determine whether surgery had benefited patients whose lives had been severely compromised by temporal lobe epilepsy. Almost half of the patients had had their temporal lobes explored (with gentle electrical stimulation), and of these 10 per cent reported experiential hallucinations.

Each patient remained conscious throughout the procedure, and was able to discuss the effect of the electrodes' application to their cortex. The surgeon then dictated the findings to a secretary who sat apart, behind a glass viewing stand.[14] The surgeons probed all the surfaces of the temporal lobe (lateral, superior, medial and inferior) and took directions from the patients. Penfield and his colleagues transcribed some of the conversations.

Case 3. – R.W. (a twelve-year-old boy whose seizures had begun three years earlier) – was one of the most fascinating. The researchers' report gave a summary of the boy's verbatim responses after the electrode repeatedly probed locations on the surface of his temporal lobe. The various regions of the temporal lobe explored were labelled from 22 to 32.

Region 22: He said nothing for a little interval, and then said, 'Oh, gee, gosh, robbers are coming at me with guns!' He heard nothing, he just saw them coming at him.
Region 23: 'Pain in my forehead, and there was a robber. He wasn't in front; he was off to the left side.'
Region 24: 'Yes, the robbers are coming after me.'
Region 28: 'Oh gosh! There they are, my brother is there. He is aiming a rifle at me.' His eyes moved slowly to the left. The figures seemed to disappear before the cessation of the stimulus.
Region 30: 'I heard someone speaking, my mother telling one of my aunts to come up tonight.'
Region 31: 'Would you do that again, please?'
Region 31: Repeated. After a pause, he said, 'The same as before. My mother was telling my aunt over the telephone to come up and visit us tonight.'

Region 32: 'My mother is telling my brother he has got his coat on backwards. I can just hear them.' When asked if he remembered it, he said, 'Oh yes, just before I came here.' When asked if he thought these things were like dreams, he said, 'No . . . it is just like I go into a daze.'

The boy's responses corresponded to the hallucinatory pattern of his epileptic attacks that had been noted at previous consultations. And now following the electrical probes and his complementary responses the neurologists mapped out and proposed a small section of the temporal lobe for surgical removal.[15]

Overall, Penfield and his researchers were surprised by the number of times music formed part of the volunteers' hallucinations; there were reports of hallelujah choirs but though a number of patients were 'aware of attendant pleasure or fear' there was no reference to a recall of any experience resembling an ecstatic one. When transported elsewhere patients were able to differentiate between the hallucinations and reality, saying things such as 'I see people in this world and that world, too.' But the range of experiences appears to have been limited. The recall of experiences, for example, did not include carrying out skilled acts, eating, suffering or sexual excitement. Penfield was at a loss as to these absences, writing that 'modesty does not explain their silences'. He speculated that the researchers might have to probe elsewhere in the cortex; that 'these things that are absent from our experiential recall may all be recorded somewhere and may be made available by other means'.[16]

Though the incidence of ecstatic auras appears to be rare, there have been sufficient anecdotal accounts over the past fifty years to galvanise scientists to continue to theorise and search for their source. In the nineteenth century, Hughlings Jackson advanced the hypothesis that the hallucinatory effects of complex mental dreamy states did not result directly from the epileptic discharge but that an alteration in consciousness came about because the regulatory/inhibitory function of the higher centres of the brain were somehow diminished in the course of the discharge, allowing for greater excitability in the lower centres.

More recently, neurologists have focused on the possible importance of religious predisposition as a determining factor in ecstatic hallucinations. And here, modesty *might* actually explain the relative silence on the part of patients, but there is also the likelihood of fear. For there are consequences in admitting to symptoms that could deliver you from treatment by a neurologist into the care of a psychiatrist. What happens when you describe symptoms that stray across the border that divides the essentially benign curiosities of some hallucinations into the pathology of psychosis? It was just such a borderland that was patrolled by researchers in 1970 who investigated 'sudden religious conversions in temporal lobe epilepsy'.

A study by Slater and Beard of the schizophrenia-like psychoses of epilepsy concluded that 'mystical delusional experiences were remarkably common'.[7] Their report included the case of a bus driver whose minor seizures had been studded by periods of automatism. During one of these attacks he departed from the regular route, drove off into some back streets and only found his way once more on the established route twenty minutes later. He'd subsequently been demoted to bus conductor. And it was whilst in the middle of collecting fares in 1955 that he was suddenly overwhelmed with a sense of heavenly bliss: 'He collected the fare correctly, telling his passengers at the same time how pleased he was to be in heaven.' He later told a doctor that he felt as though a 'bomb had burst in his head' ... He was constantly laughing to himself ... He remained in this state of exaltation, hearing divine and angelic voices, for two days.' God had granted the conductor a one-way ticket to heaven and he pitied those who remained stuck on earth.

Over the next two years the bus conductor retained his religious fervour but then in 1958, after three successive seizures, 'he became elated again and said his mind had "cleared" . . . During this episode he lost his faith' and had a sudden, revelatory re-conversion to agnosticism.

If these conversions and re-conversions were a consequence of ecstatic hallucinations, then what was their trigger? When Penfield and his colleagues were able to provoke experiential illusions with the electrode probes, they were, of course, reliant on the subjective responses of the patients to confirm that that was the case. But just over a decade ago, researchers employed even more subtle and less invasive means to try independently to measure the activity of the brain contiguous with ecstatic auras.

Embarking on a novel approach in researching temporal lobe epilepsy, a behavioural neurobiologist, Vilayanur Ramachandran, compared people with and without the condition. He measured galvanic skin responses to visual stimuli, namely how much the volunteers sweated when exposed to different types of imagery. Much to his amazement, Ramachandran found that 'every time they [the temporal lobe patients] looked at religious words like God they'd get a huge galvanic skin response'. Ramachandran concluded that the stimuli had activated specific neural circuits that were more prone to religious beliefs. It was a radical and controversial finding. Vilayanur Ramachandran further explored the connection between so-called 'God spot' seizures and the irritability and obsessive-compulsive behaviour also associated with temporal lobe epilepsy. But he came no closer than any predecessor to more specifically locating the so-called spot in the brain where a feeling for God is said to exist.

In more recent years researchers such as the neurologist Fabienne Picard have turned their attention to the insula as a possible candidate for the God spot. This is a small region buried in a fissure separating the frontal and parietal lobes from the temporal lobes. When the brains of volunteers with temporal lobe epilepsy were imaged during seizures (with an injection of nuclear traces) the scans later revealed an increase in the blood flow to the insula – suggesting hyperactivity in that area and a rise in the level of neurotransmitters. This is akin to the increase in the levels of serotonin known to accompany the ingestion of ecstasy tablets. And when subsequently another group of patients had electrode probes inserted to stimulate the insula, the patients described feelings of well-being and ecstasy similar to those recorded by Penfield.

Listening to her patients describing their experiences, Picard attempted to classify the ecstatic auras, dividing them into three broad categories: hyper-consciousness; an increased sense of well-being; and a spiritual sense of harmony. During these moments patients often also spoke of time slowing down (in the way that has been noted by people who have been involved, for example, in car accidents).

Picard suggested that prediction error might account for the feelings of harmony. The theory of prediction error states that there is an area of the brain that anticipates our sense of an experience and then compares it to the actual (realised) sense. If the result (the actual sense) is close to the predicted sense then we are left with a feeling of well-being. But if the actual sense is far apart from that which is predicted then it leads to anxiety. This further directed research into the insula, in particular to the front part of the insula which is thought to be responsible for emotions and bodily awareness.

The insula works in this way by selecting sensations at startling speeds of 125 milliseconds which some scholars have labelled 'global moments'. During the increased excitation of ecstatic auras the insula samples these salami-slices of global moments at such enhanced speeds that patients have the feeling of experience slowed down. It is reminiscent of the tale of the 'no-time' of the Prophet Muhammad's celestial vision. As Muhammad's vision began a jug of water was knocked over, but before the water spilled from the jug Muhammad had been transported to Paradise and back again.

The notion that people with epilepsy have a special quality, that they can act as conduits between this world and the next, is alive in many cultures. Throw out that suggestion into the wind and it will return with interest, whether it is reflections on Joan of Arc and the Prophet Muhammad, the Siberian physicians who in past centuries expressed a preference for pupils with epilepsy because of their alleged mystical powers,[18] or the reverence shown towards people with epilepsy by the Hmong of Laos. In *The Spirit Catches You and You Fall Down*, Anne Fadiman recounted the commonly held view amongst the Hmong people that the whole family felt blessed if a member turned out to have epilepsy – it was a condition of distinction often identified with shamans selected for the healing spirit because of their high moral character.[19]

But for all of the suggestions of special privileges for epilepsy there is a welter of disadvantages to contend with; and might not the patients' hyper-religiosity be a consequence of the condition, and simply act as a welcome and necessary balm to offset the daily injuries and insults? If epilepsy is an old and familiar but unwanted friend who arrives unbidden and who doesn't so much as doff his cap, before barging into your life, then how does your relationship change with it as you age?

It did not make my brother more brittle, as I expected. In those earlier angry years when the epileptic fix was on, in the midst of the strange exaggerated hiccupping I felt he was trying to resist its claim on him. But with age, he seemed to grow more accepting, as if he had reached some accommodation with the seizures. At times he woke after a seizure with a look of such disappointment;

and I imagined him at the end of a dialogue with the fits urging them not to go just yet, like Horatio commanding the ghost of King Hamlet, 'Stay, illusion!'

If Christopher became more mysterious with age and surrendered to mysticism, it was but for a moment. The mysticism always passed into stoicism. And I have seen the same countless times in others with epilepsy.

In epilepsy's ledger of credits and deficits, what is to be found on the credits side? Is there really anything to be gained from epilepsy? Is there anything that an epileptic might miss if a cure was available tomorrow? Scores of liberated slaves, African Americans, who travelled the Underground Railroad with Harriet Tubman, inadvertently owe their freedom to the slave owner who struck Tubman over the head, bequeathing her a lifetime of headaches and visions from temporal lobe epilepsy. Might not Harriet Tubman have mourned the loss of those visions following brain surgery in later life to relieve her incessant head troubles? And would temporal lobe epileptics trade their heightened religiosity and supernatural experiences for a more equitable, vision-free life?

In reviewing historical cases, it's important to question the degree to which physicians might have been aware of the possibility of false visions or holy madness being the consequence of epilepsy. Mark Salzman set out to explore just such a premise in his novel *Lying Awake*. The Carmelite nun at the centre of the book has for almost thirty years been cloistered away from the trappings of modern life. She suffers terrible, searing headaches but is also exalted by ecstatic auras which allow her to commune with God. In her transcendent state she is likened to 'an ember carried upward by the heat of an invisible flame'. The author delves into centuries-long debate over false visions and holy madness. But when it transpires that the visions are the result of a tumour on her temporal lobe she is confronted with a dilemma. Removing the tumour will cure her of the debilitating headaches but it will also close her portal to God.

Just such a dilemma was further investigated in a small Norwegian survey completed a decade ago which also sought to determine whether it mattered that epiphanic visions had a biological root, when they served a private passion. Asheim and Brodtkorb tested eleven people with epilepsy who had complex sensory seizures, in which 'eight had sensory hallucinations, four had erotic sensations, five described "a religious/spiritual experience", and several had symptoms that were felt to have no counterpart in human experience'.

The first patient described how difficult it was to resist the 'trance of pleasure' of the hallucination: 'It is like an emotional wave striking me again and again. I feel compelled to obey a sort of phenomenon of the fit taking control.' Not only was he unable to resist, however, he also admitted feeling addicted to his auras.

Crucially, the researchers found that the majority would have welcomed a repeat of the sometimes spiritual experiences of the seizure. Several confided that they were so delighted by the 'woolly' feeling that they tried to induce a seizure later on so that the feeling would be repeated, for instance by recalling the smell of sawdust that had accompanied the aura, or by reducing the dose of their anti-epileptic medication. More than one described the auras as a guilty pleasure for which they would subsequently be punished with unpleasant headaches and nausea.

One patient who had been free of seizures for a while nostalgically yearned their passing as adults do their youth: 'Nowadays I sometimes miss the attacks,' she said. 'They gave me feelings I thought I was too old to experience.'

Certainly Fyodor Dostoevsky would have been in their camp. He cherished his rare ecstatic seizures and would have us believe that epileptics as well as the meek would inherit the earth. During those glorified moments, Dostoevsky confided to his friend the philosopher and critic Nikolay Strakhov that before the onset of an attack there were minutes in which he was in rapture: 'For several moments,' he said, 'I would experience such joy as would be inconceivable in ordinary life – such joy that no one else could have any notion of. I would feel the most complete harmony in myself and in the whole world and this feeling was so strong and sweet that for a few seconds of such bliss I would give ten or more years of my life, even my whole life perhaps.'

In the photograph Christopher stands, hands in pockets, alone in the grounds of Micklepage, the fourteenth-century farmhouse and retreat that Jo and I hired for our wedding in 2002. Christopher stares at the camera with steady but misty eyes – not from the emotion of the wedding; that is yet to come.

My brother has a thick plaster over his forehead. It is dark, stained purple where some blood is still seeping through. His misty eyes contain the detritus of a seizure that he has had an hour before. We had hoped that the epilepsy would grant him a day off from the fits on our wedding day, but we suspected it would not; that there would be no let-up.

I recall now the story beyond the borders of that photograph; how Christopher caught me staring at him with concern; how he approached me with a big beaming smile and whispered, 'Don't let it spoil your day. You will remember this day.'

And I do remember it now, not for the upsetting, sad start to the wedding but for the revelatory and ecstatic end to an extraordinarily emotional and exhausting day.

Close to midnight, half a dozen of us, the last of the revellers, gathered around the long kitchen table, drawing the celebrations to a close. The mood was convivial, but there was something peculiar about my place in that setting. All around me I could see animated lips moving and throats swelling with laughter, but I could not hear anything. All was still and quiet. And, for a moment, no more, I was suddenly overcome with a feeling and a thought of absolute clarity that life was going to be 'just so' – not only here and now but in the future; and that it was always going to be thus; that I need not have worried in the past; that those years of anxiety and struggle were insignificant and were never going to count, for everything had been a preparation for this moment of exaltation.

I struggled to describe the feeling to the group. Some laughed and suggested the influence of marijuana; but then Christopher began to speak, and his words were like a continuation of my own. Uncannily, it was as if he was describing exactly that which could only have been known to me. When I looked at him in wonder for an explanation, Christopher answered, 'Yes, I know that feeling. Beautiful, isn't it? I've been to that other place. Been there. Done it.'

'When?'

'During one of my thingamajigs,' said Christopher.

'Thingamajigs?'

'Yes.'

'Is that what we're calling them now?'

Christopher didn't answer. He was falling into his own reverie.

'How many times have you had it – that feeling?' I asked.

'Oh, not enough,' said Christopher. 'Not nearly enough.'

And I often wondered subsequently over the years, on the few occasions when Christopher zoned out momentarily in a conversation from a minor seizure and was restored to full consciousness with what looked like an expression of bliss, whether he had travelled to that other place. I hoped so.

Bad Brain is Worse than No Brain

At about three o'clock in the morning there was a knock on the front door. Given the hour, it was not as timid or as apologetic as might have been expected. But then neither was it fervent or demanding. If anything it was speculative. I pulled the door open. A tall policeman in a blue-black uniform filled the frame of the doorway. He said my name, nothing more. People's language in the early hours tends to be economical; and A&E staff, night porters and the police are, it seems, especially versed in linguistic minimalism. 'Colin Grant?' asked the policeman again. I nodded. He half-turned and gestured back to the car: 'We've got something of yours, I believe.'

I could just make out a figure, sitting on the back seat of the police car. The door sprang open like a trap, and my brother stepped out gingerly; he was barefooted.

'What's happened to his shoes?' I asked the taciturn police constable.

'I couldn't really say, sir.'

'You don't know, or you'd rather not say?'

'I couldn't really say, sir.'

He volunteered little else other than to repeat the verbal warning he'd already given Christopher after they'd found him walking along the side of the motorway. That fact and the missing shoes were not so much of an enigma to me. Most often any bizarre behaviour displayed by Christopher was associated with his epilepsy, and was an indication that he had probably lapsed yet again in taking his medication.

'If he would just tek the medicine. Why the boy can't tek the medicine, God for tell,' was a constant refrain of my mother's.

When questioned about his non-compliance Christopher would counter that the drugs didn't work or that they dulled him and left him thick-headed. Other sufferers have spoken about how they have felt trapped in this way by the condition. The seizures themselves can leave them feeling that their very consciousness is diminished and dulled; and so, too, can the prescribed medication. The difference for Christopher was that with a seizure that dullness was acute and finite; with the drugs it was constant and chronic. Straight after a big attack and subjected to a chorus of nagging from us, Christopher was liable to agree to take the medication but then a week later, in that phoney period between one seizure and the next, he'd default to a more cavalier attitude and announce that he was taking a chemical sabbatical.

The huge number of remedies devised for epilepsy over the centuries reflected the fact that they rarely proved of lasting benefit: in the end, they didn't work. Up until the nineteenth century the treatment of epilepsy had been hampered by a fundamental misunderstanding about its pathology. The latter half of that century was a particularly fertile period for experimentation, and the search for the drug that would settle the matter became a kind of Holy Grail. For the very first physician appointed at the National Hospital, Jabez Spence Ramskill, it was an obsession. Not a week passed without him bringing to the laboratory 'a specimen of a new drug, always hopeful that he had found in it a cure for epilepsy'. Unfortunately, thirty-five years after he had embarked on his unending inquiry into drug treatment, Ramskill died, neither having completed nor published his long-awaited report.[1]

Largely though, medical expertise in the treatment of the condition was still anecdotal and no more rigorous than old wives' tales. Popularly, a solid constitution was said to serve as the primary bedrock in the fight against epilepsy. In the Goulstonian lectures on epilepsy in 1860, for example, Charles Bland Radcliffe championed a common-sense twofold approach: a modest intake of alcohol ('unquestionable good will result from a proper allowance of sherry, weak brandy-and-water, or better still, of claret'); and regular familiarity with the chamber pot ('the avoidance of constipation and the accumulation of effete matters in the bowels'.) Even William Gowers agreed on this latter point: 'In all cases it is most desirable that regular action of the bowels should be secured. Nothing conduces to the occurrence of attacks more than constipation and gastric disturbance.'[2]

When their contemporary, the eminent neurologist Sir Edward Sieveking, conducted a survey of his own practice, he listed an extraordinary array of prescriptions, including myriad salts, indigo, preparations of silver, zinc and bromide. And reviewing the claims made by proponents of epileptic cures, Sieveking observed (without sarcasm), 'There is scarcely a substance in the world, capable of passing through the gullet of man, that has not at one time or other enjoyed a reputation of being an anti-epileptic.'[3]

He was right. So it was from the very beginning of man's intervention in the progress of epilepsy. Imagine the most bizarre and unlikely remedy for epilepsy and it's probably already been tried. As a potential cure few can have surpassed the ancient Roman custom of draining the blood from the severed head of a gladiator and drinking it. Stiff competition, though, came from concoctions believed to have other occult qualities, including extracts from sparrow's brains, bear's testicles and the stomachs of hares.[4]

Always there was the search for a wonder drug or miracle cure, and a strong belief in the curative power of nature. For many centuries, root of peony was the primary remedy of choice amongst serious physicians. Galen's experience was often cited as a precedent; and had the power of celebrity endorsement. The Galenic approach to medicine was revered and adhered to more than a thousand years after his death. The Roman master physician had famously and excitedly recounted a case of juvenile epilepsy which was arrested when a boy wore an amulet (of root of peony) around his neck, but Galen noted, 'When, however, somehow, the amulet slid off, he was immediately seized.' To prove the connection Galen then 'hung a big, fresh part of the root around his neck. And from that time on the boy was healthy and was no longer seized by convulsions.'

Galen's apparent enthusiasm for peony came with doctorly caveats and caution: 'I do not entirely relinquish the hope,' he wrote, 'that it may have been reasonable to rely on it to cure epilepsy in children.'[5] Even so, the plant's virtues were still being praised into the seventeenth century when the influential and radical apothecary and astrologer Nicholas Culpeper, though he carried no brief for Galen, advocated the root of the male peony as a 'cure for falling sickness' in adults 'if the disease be not grown too old and past cure'. There were a number of ways, according to Culpeper, in which the medicine could be administered but the surest method was to make an infusion that should be taken before and after a full moon.[6]

Culpeper unnerved the Establishment by stressing both the medicinal virtues and astrological properties of his remedies. But his underlying intention was to promote a kind of medical egalitarianism giving the poor access to knowledge and the tools to cure themselves. Fundamentally, Nicholas Culpeper understood that a patient's belief in the treatment made it more effective. What apothecaries such as Culpeper really provided was an infusion of hope.[7]

If conflict over corporeal control and order raged, as it did in Culpeper's time, between medical practitioners (physicians and apothecaries); then so too in the twenty-first century have physicians become alarmed by the shift in the relationship with patients who challenge their authority. Early on at medical school we were guided by the new, invigorating principle and language of holistic medicine (to attend to the patient's physical and spiritual well-being). I say 'new' but the same philosophy underpinned the views of the neurologist William Aldren Turner, who in 1910 was counselling against the reliance of medicinal means in the treatment of epilepsy, because there was the need 'in every case of epilepsy to treat the individual and not solely the disease'.[8] All too often in their dealings with Christopher, a century on from Turner, the medics lost faith in the idealism of a holistic approach and worse still, somewhere between the words 'first' and 'do no harm' of the Hippocratic oath their moral compass seemed to go awry. They could not understand him, nor he them.

Once I sat in on a GP's consultation with Christopher who in attempting to explain his antipathy towards the drugs introduced the notion of Koyaanisqatsi, the Native American Hopi word meaning 'life out of balance'. The medication reduced him; it left him with a feeling, he said, of living a life out of sync or out of harmony, as explored in his favourite film with that same name, *Koyaanisqatsi*.

'Do you see?' asked Christopher. The GP's thoughts were elsewhere. He did not respond. My brother sat forward now – the better to give himself some room – and slowly bellowed in a deep rumbling voice, 'Koyaanisqatsi,' imitating the chant of a Hopi elder: '*Koyaanisqatsi. Koyaanisqatsi.*'

The GP looked up from the computer screen where he'd been transcribing Christopher's complaint. He hadn't met Christopher before. 'What dose of sodium valproate are you on?'

'Five hundred milligrams,' said Christopher.

'Five hundred?'

'Yes.'

'Mmmh.'

I imagined the GP's superior 'mmmh' signalled his disagreement with what had been prescribed; but 'mmmh' would be as far as he would go in criticising a colleague.

He started to scribble on the prescription pad. 'I think we could tweak that dose. You're feeling a little out of sorts, you say?'

'No, out of sync,' insisted Christopher.

'Well, not taking the medication,' said the GP drily, 'will leave you feeling even more out of sorts.'

Whilst Christopher viewed his non-compliance with anti-epileptic drugs as self-protection, the GPs and other medics judged it as injurious to him and wilfully self-inflicted. In some sense both were right.

But Christopher was not alone. The same can be said of Neil Young, Ian Curtis and myriad others. Their narrative of disenchantment has been repeated down the years with the arrival of every new wonder drug, and the initial faith which both parties (doctors and patients) place in it. Not until the nineteenth century would the first universally approved remedy arrive. Before then people with epilepsy were subjected to the kind of common futile practices such as bloodletting which would have caused the radical apothecaries to roll their eyes.

Two hundred years on from Culpeper, bloodletting was still regularly employed as preventative therapy and for the amelioration of epilepsy. A nineteenth-century diary would reveal just how sufferers, and those charged with draining off the blood, steeled themselves to that which they considered a necessary inhumanity.

Between 1829 and 1834, W. Silke of Mistley in Essex kept a diary of his wife's illnesses and symptoms.[9]

March 31st, 1830 . . . This Morning about half past ten my dearest Wife was again seized with dreadful convulsion fits which continued till after four—Mr. Thompson abstracted about six or eight ounces of Blood by cupping between the Shoulders.

Occasionally she would need to 'have her Head shaved' (for cupping).

July 19th, 1830 . . . This Morning about ten o Clock . . . another fit . . . lasted at least half an hour—As soon as She partly recovered her senses, She submitted to be Cupped, and bore the operation with exemplary fortitude, considering how many times her dear Head and Back have been scarified.

On 15 August 1830, 'in hopes of preventing a recurrence of Epilepsy', cupping was again employed, siphoning off 'about half a pound of Blood'.

On 26 and 29 December 1832, Silke's diary records frequent 'flushings of the face accompanied with a full pulse and great excitement' or 'nervous irritation' prompting the removal of 8 ounces of blood by cupping on 26 December. Five days later, she had the 'slightest fit' and hoped the cupping had mitigated its severity.

Mrs Silke's condition continued to decline after a severe seizure in October 1833. She had 'slight' fits on 11 February, 2 April, and 12 May 1834. She died on 25 June 1834.

Up until the 1800s there had been no standardised treatment for epilepsy; and no real agreement. Physicians were no better placed than the layman or woman in treating epilepsy. 'If any old woman had the possession of a herb or a salt which could antagonise the disease [epilepsy],' observed Sir Samuel Wilks, 'the knowledge would be worth more than that of the whole College of Physicians.'[10]

But in the latter half of the nineteenth century a kind of consensus arose amongst these so-called ignorant physicians in Europe and the Americas with the introduction of a simple salt, a soluble white crystalline powder, potassium bromide, which would be hailed as a wonder drug. Initially, though, there was no great fanfare for the introduction of bromide as a drug that might prove effective in suppressing epileptic fits. Rather, bromide appeared in the margins, as it were, in the discussions that followed an important presentation on epilepsy at the Royal Medical and Chirurgical Society in London in May 1857. Sir Charles Locock, a famous obstetrician who presided over the meeting, reviewing more than fifty cases of epilepsy, astonished delegates when he revealed, almost as an afterthought, that he'd tried out a new remedy; he had administered potassium bromide to a patient whom he described as suffering from 'hysterical epilepsy'.[11] Physicians had been perplexed by these kinds of seizures which, though closely resembling epileptic attacks, did not result from any pathological, electrical discharge in the brain; they were thought to be particularly prevalent in women, were suspected by some to emanate from the uterus, and appeared to occur more often when witnesses were present.

Locock had been drawn to bromide after reading a report by a German researcher who'd experimented with the drug on himself. Over the course of a fortnight, the physician had taken ten grains of a bromide preparation three times a day and found that it temporarily caused impotence: 'the virile powers returning after leaving off the medicine'. Locock immediately saw its potential as a cure for a condition the German physician might not have imagined: hysterical epilepsy.

For almost a decade, Charles Locock had been baffled by his inability effectively to treat a patient who'd regularly attended his clinic with signs and symptoms of hysterical epilepsy. Nothing had worked. The patient's condition was exacerbated by her menstrual cycle, and deemed a manifestation of her heightened 'sexual excitement'. She was an ideal candidate, thought Locock, for the new salt. His reasoning was simple. Hysteria in unmarried young women was thought to be triggered by sexual excitement and was widely believed, at that time, to be calmed by marriage. Locock hoped that bromide might serve just as well as a husband. And it did. He was delighted to report to colleagues that since taking potassium bromide the woman had had no subsequent attacks of hysterical epilepsy. He then tried the remedy on another fifteen women, with remarkable success, allegedly, in all but one of the patients. Modern researchers have cast doubt on the feasibility of Charles Locock's assertion and the high rate of his success but the medical profession needs to take his word on the matter for Locock declined to publish the details of his findings. In any event, there would have been no call back in 1857 to question the integrity of one of the most fashionable gentleman physicians who listed the Queen amongst his clientele.[12]

Sir Charles Locock's testimony was only part of a response he'd given as president of the Royal Medical and Chirurgical Society; he'd also called on his colleagues not to overlook the fact that in boys and girls masturbation was often a cause of epilepsy. Whilst there was agreement among delegates that this was frequently the case, particularly 'in the southern climates', the requisite delicacy when treating females made it near impossible to definitively determine masturbation as a causal effect. Nonetheless, the firmly held belief in the link fuelled late-nineteenth-century physicians' advocacy of castration as a cure for some forms of juvenile epilepsy.[13] Locock need hardly have spelt out the conclusion that masturbatory boys and girls might benefit from the less invasive treatment of bromide. And in the coming years other doctors made a further speculative leap in prescribing bromide for patients whose epilepsy was non-hysterical. The results, they claimed, were similarly impressive.

A handful of studies carried out in England and the USA backed up Locock's findings – though the results were far more modest. Researchers at Northampton's lunatic asylum in 1864, for instance, reported a reduction by a fifth in the numbers of seizures suffered by inmates after bromide therapy.[14] William Aldred Turner reported similar results – long-term remission was seen in a quarter of the 366 cases under his care.[15] For those who benefited, it must indeed have seemed a miracle drug. But bromide's real rise was built on the back of a number of prominent cheerleaders, amongst them Charles Bland Radcliffe. Though he wasn't sure how and why it worked, Dr Radcliffe began to prescribe it 'almost promiscuously' and trumpeted, 'Bromide potassium is the only remedy in epilepsy upon which most dependence can be placed.' It surely heralded, wrote Radcliffe, 'a brighter future in the fortunes of epileptics', thanks to Sir Charles's intervention.[16]

At the National Hospital, the ever vigilant Ramskill was an early adopter of bromide therapy and William Gowers, too, was an enthusiast. In his important book on epilepsy Gowers devoted a chapter to treatment in which he noted that bromide had 'almost superseded other drugs in the treatment for the disease'. He conceded that its influence was largely transient. After all, there were two major drawbacks: for bromide to be effective it needed continuous administration of small doses; if you overdid the dosage it would put the patient to sleep. Bromides, it turned out, had 'a direct effect on the nerve elements, diminishing for instance, reflex action in the spinal cord'. And one unfortunate consequence of this direct action on the nerve cells of the brain was 'mental dullness and somnolence'.[17]

Nonetheless, by the end of the century, 2.5 tons of bromide were being dispensed by the pharmacy at the National Hospital – a huge amount, the equivalent of 3,000 patient-years of treatment. The scale of bromide's use was also mirrored elsewhere in Europe and the USA, and proved profitable for manufacturers. The pharmacy of the Bethel epileptic colony, for example, made a handsome return on its exports of the drug. The profits would have been greater but for its internal market. Bethel itself consumed vast amounts, as bromide was doled out daily to the colonists, on whom the two most obvious properties unrelated to its anti-epileptic potential were considered by some staff to be a bonus. Not only did bromide appear to reduce the number of seizures on the mixed population of colonists, but it also reduced their sex drive and served as a somnolent pacifier. Staff would have difficulty squaring this latter effect with the stated philosophy of Bethel to enable colonists to lead fuller lives through physical occupation.

More worryingly, a decade after the introduction of bromide treatment some physicians such as Samuel Wilks were beginning to question its long-term benefits; he alleged that bromide suppressed but did not cure, and that mitigation was not enough; for some patients, Wilks believed, are 'greatly relieved after an explosive fit has taken place and feel worse if it has been prevented, as if some injurious force within them were struggling to get free'. In such instances the seizure almost acted as a purge, in the way that a sickly person's nausea might be purged through vomiting. Wilks went on to voice the thankfully not so common complaint of 'other epileptics who say they would rather have the fits than undergo the unpleasant sensations which from time to time seem to be substituted for them'.[18]

Wilks was referring to the increasing number of patients who were turning up at clinics and describing disturbing signs and symptoms that would later be attributed to excessive consumption of the bromide salt, and were a consequence of its 'promiscuous' prescription.

The symptoms included memory loss, slowing of speech, a never-ending flow of saliva, unsteady movements, flatulence, diarrhoea, nausea and, most distressingly for some, an eruption of acne on the skin of the face and back.[19] The symptoms were sufficiently repetitive and so obviously derived from a single source to warrant a name. This then was the catch: the treatment of one condition, epilepsy, spawned another condition, bromism.

Today it is recognised that as little as 0.5 grams of bromide can lead to bromism. But over a century ago, doctors were prescribing ten times that amount. The large doses were thought to be required to reach a threshold at which seizures might be arrested; the problem was further compounded by the very long half-life of bromide which meant that it took a long time to decay, so that toxic levels of the drug accumulated in the body.

By 1900 the fervour that had accompanied and surrounded bromide began to dampen down. 'Many are yearly declaring against it [bromide therapy],' wrote L. P. Clark. 'Its abuse has grown great, and the routine treatment of all cases by bromides is not only poor therapy, but actual culpable negligence.'[20]

Doctors have a reputation for conservatism but in their use of bromide many were cavalier – if not callous. As the neurologist Simon Shorvon has observed, 'Bromides were often used in punitive dosages by physicians who cared little about the physical and mental damage wreaked by the drug.'[21]

The known side effects did not lead to a diminution of the drug's rate of prescription. The figures were astonishing. It took a few decades before the dangers were universally recognised, so much so that by 1928, in the US 20 per cent of all prescriptions written by physicians were for bromides.[22] The popularity of the drug outstripped its control when it became – as it did in the USA – readily available 'over the counter' without the need for a doctor's approval.

Happenstance had led to the discovery and rise of bromide when in 1857 the Queen's accoucheur alighted on an obscure German paper. In 1912 serendipity was also to lead to the emergence of a rival drug when a junior hospital doctor, on call overnight, was made irritable through sleep deprivation. In an account that has now crossed over into medical history legend, Alfred Hauptmann was trying and failing to sleep each night in the doctors' rooms above a ward in a clinic in Freiburg. He couldn't sleep because of being disturbed by patients who kept him awake with their nocturnal epileptic seizures. Hauptmann reasoned that if the patients could be sedated during the night he might have a chance to catch up on his own sleep. He gave them phenobarbital (Luminal), a recently synthesised drug prescribed as a hypnotic and sedative, and his own sleep was successfully restored. But then Hauptmann observed that not only did phenobarbital quieten the patients; it curbed their noisy seizures as well. Hauptmann followed up this accidental discovery, selecting patients with chronic epilepsy (who'd been resistant to bromide therapy) and prescribing them phenobarbital instead. Over the course of several months and years of adjusting and tweaking the doses, Hauptmann worked out that phenobarbital could also successfully arrest seizures in even less severe cases of patients with epilepsy, and with fewer adverse effects than bromide. Another miracle cure had been born.

German patients, however, remained the sole beneficiaries for longer than would have been expected, primarily because the outbreak of the First World War hindered the prescription of phenobarbital elsewhere. In Britain it would not be administered until 1920, long after hostilities had ceased. Thereafter its uptake was widespread and within a decade almost universal. It might have continued in this vein but for one disturbing fact (as far as the manufacturers were concerned): it was cheap.

The next major drug, most commonly used after phenobarbital, from the late 1930s onwards, was phenytoin. Championed by an advocate in the journal *Epilepsia*, phenytoin was said to be 'more effective than phenobarbital in stopping the various types of seizures, and is without the depressive effect on the mentality'. But all pharmacological treatments have had deleterious side effects (phenytoin included) that discouraged patients from taking them. The same is as true today as it was in the 1930s.

The dilemma of drug compliance versus non-compliance resonates with the writer M who, now in his early sixties, was diagnosed with epilepsy as a teenager. Back then he was forced to curb some of his activities, but even so the fits continued: 'After A levels I was of the group that was expected to apply for Oxford and Cambridge and expected to go there. But in that extra term I did no work; I could not work at all. I did not go to Cambridge. And one of the shocking things was that I had been a sort of golden boy. And yet I never heard from the school again.'[23]

M was not reconciled to a life on medication but he reached a stage where the dangers were becoming too alarming; when for instance he managed to pull a pan of boiling water over himself.

'The more specialists I saw the more drugs they wanted me to take but I simply didn't want to do that because I already felt a bit obtunded and it only was when the effects of the very frequent fits exceeded the side effects of the drugs [that I relented].'

For all that has befallen him, M is surprisingly a prodigious smiler with lambent eyes that invite you into the warmth of his world. He is an attentive and gracious intellectual and yet seems to exist permanently on the edge of amusement, laughing all the way through our discussion. Sanguine now about his own epileptic past, M still occasionally mourns his brighter self:

'There was a time when I enjoyed my brain. I felt it was sharp and my professional life at that stage, such as it was, required me to have a sharp brain, but now . . . You know when you wake up with a hangover and the first thing you've got to do is push your way through that thickness of cotton wool to get to where you can operate but actually that bit there [the sharpness] that's gone – you can't get to that point.'

There are strategies that M can use to compensate for the limitations of both the medication and the epilepsy. But a bigger compensation perhaps is that because of the drugs, he has been free from fits for two decades, living in an age of medical materialism 'with neurophysiology, electrophysiology, biochemistry and pharmacology all on my side'.

The daily dose of anti-convulsants, the pink Smartie-like Epilim tablets, is of course a lot more attractive than the cornucopia of remedies and treatments that would have been his lot in the past – the application of a ligature, compression of the carotid arteries, sexual abstinence, wearing herbal amulets, avoidance of contact with goats, drinking the blood from the head of a decapitated gladiator, injecting rattlesnake venom and of course, trepanning.

In modern times remedies included psychoanalysis. Up until the first half of the twentieth century there was still a lively debate about whether epilepsy was a neurological condition or a psychiatric illness. Fyodor Dostoevsky was a case in point. As previously mentioned, Freud considered hysteria to be the basis of Dostoevsky's seizures.

The attention given to hysterical epilepsy now seems like a false turn in the history of medicine. Today, it would be considered inappropriate for any practitioner to suggest analysis as a course of treatment for epilepsy. But older forms of therapy that might seem as peculiar and primitive have never disappeared. Brain surgery might appear relatively modern but its earliest manifestation, trepanation, dates back at least to the thirteenth century when the surgical text *Quattuor Magistri* suggested opening the skulls of melancholics, epileptics and others, 'that the humours and airs may go out and evapourate'.[24] Trepanning was still considered an option in 1970 when the writer M had his first epileptic fit. The then sixteen-year-old M had blacked out on an overnight ferry to Hamburg. Soon after his return to England, early on in his diagnosis, it was suggested to his parents that he might benefit from trepanning. They were alarmed about the prospect of a surgeon drilling holes into their adolescent son's head and, thankfully, says M, sought another opinion. But he continues to be haunted by the memory of that close shave, and to wonder, What if? What if he'd lived in a different age? How would things have turned out?

Forty years earlier he might very well have been offered surgery. The 1930s witnessed revolutionary and controversial advances as innovative surgical procedures appeared to offer some hope for those whose epilepsy was resistant to drugs.

Modern neurosurgery has its roots in the radical work of the previously mentioned Wilder Penfield who in the mid-1930s, having migrated from the USA to Canada, pioneered a technique which became known as the Montreal procedure. Under his care, patients with severe epilepsy deemed eligible for surgery were given a local anaesthetic but remained fully conscious while he operated. Penfield then removed a section of the skull cap to expose the brain tissue. As the surgeon electrically probed the brain, the patient would describe his feelings up to the point where the stimulation appeared to replicate the sense of seizure activity, so that Penfield could then map that specific site on the cortex of the brain. That 'bad' brain tissue was subsequently removed. And post-operatively the epileptic seizures would cease – at least that was the working theory. The hundreds of patients who volunteered for the Montreal procedure recognised that in some sense they were subjects of a pioneering clinical trial – not without its risks.

'Removal of very large areas of the human brain in neurosurgical practice offers an opportunity for detailed neurological study,' wrote Wilder Penfield in a seminal paper in 1935, 'especially in the occasional case which fortuitously presents many of the conditions which would be demanded of a physiological experiment.'[25] Wilder Penfield's frank admission should not be mistaken for a surgeon's glee or enthusiasm when presented with complex patient histories to advance medical knowledge, but it was all the more remarkable because one of the 'occasional cases' Penfield alluded to and whom he was to describe in that paper was his sister.

By 1935 Penfield was already celebrated for his skill with the scalpel and electrical probes; for his exploration and mapping of the brain as well as for his humanism. To those who were close to him, it was apparent that Penfield was motivated in part by the plight of his sister Ruth, who early on in his career underwent surgery (at his hands) after years of debilitating epileptic Jacksonian seizures.

When the sickly forty-three-year-old Ruth ventured across the border and turned up at her brother's house in Montreal in 1928 at the behest of (and accompanied by) their anxious mother, she was immediately examined by Wilder Penfield who discovered to his dismay that she had a brain tumour, an oligodendroglioma. The tumour had in all likelihood been slowly growing throughout her early adulthood (she'd only had four major seizures in two decades). But in the last few years the number of seizures had multiplied. Penfield's mother had, in desperation, sought the counsel of Christian Science, 'under the misconception that the cause was something that could be controlled by the mind'.[26] Now the tumour was malignant and aggressive: Ruth's condition was very dangerous, and the prognosis poor.

Urged on by neurosurgical colleagues, on 11 December 1928 Wilder Penfield carried out a craniotomy on his sister in preparation for amputating a section of the frontal lobe where the tumour had grown. This was the first time he had embarked on a technique picked up from German surgeons using local anaesthetic only. It was a gruelling six-hour session. Ruth remained conscious throughout except briefly, towards the end of the operation, when Penfield daringly (ignoring a colleague who warned, 'Don't chance it!') attempted to remove the last stubborn remnants of the tumour buried deep in the mesial frontal region, and 'there was a sharp haemorrhage'. Another who witnessed the procedure described it less coyly as 'massive bleeding'.[27]

Ruth survived the operation and was even apologetic for the difficulties she had caused. She was grateful that her life had been spared (so that she could mother her six children again); and was thrilled to be able to delight in the simple pleasures of life – to be welcomed back to her home, as she was later to write, by the meadowlarks and mockingbirds. There was always a chance, though, as the rump of a tumour remained, that the symptoms would return; and so it proved. Penfield asked Harvey Cushing to conduct a follow-up operation two years later but that too was unsuccessful and within a few more months Ruth died.

The death of his sister would weigh on Penfield's conscience throughout the rest of his life; he struggled to make sense of it in an autobiography which would be posthumously published, in which he confessed, 'The resentment I felt because of my inability to save my sister spurred me on to make my first bid for an endowed neurological institute.'[28] And when the surgeon considered the wisdom of writing up her case in 1935, the rationale that

Ruth's experience might be pressed into the service of science overrode any emotional timidity that her sibling had in exposing her story.

'My instinctive reaction was to withhold this case from publication,' admitted Penfield, 'but the close bond of sympathy that had existed between us makes it possible for me to evaluate the effect of the loss of the frontal lobe upon her personality and her mental capacity.' Dr Penfield thought that 'if she were alive I am sure she would approve of such an analysis in the hope that it might help others'.

Wilder Penfield was convinced that the key to understanding and treating many of the patients who presented with intractable epilepsy was to identify the cells responsible for the scar tissue which had developed after damage to their brains. Though scar formation was a healing response to trauma, the scar was also the origin of the abnormal electrical activity in the brain during seizures. Penfield had learnt from the German neurosurgeon Otfrid Foerster a technique for excising the scar tissue from the brains of people with epilepsy and applied that method at his Montreal Neurological Institute when it opened in the 1930s. In subsequent years Wilder Penfield performed hundreds of such operations, perfecting the Montreal procedure, all the while humbly reminding anyone who cared to listen that his success was based on a team effort.

At the opening of a 1960s BBC documentary focusing on the then renowned Montreal Neurological Institute (MNI), Wilder Penfield is shown in the viewing gallery above the surgical theatre. In a dark three-piece suit Dr Penfield appears more avuncular than patrician as he peers down, looking through the glass ceiling of the operating theatre, occasionally with the benefit of opera binoculars. He radiates a proud beneficence on his junior colleagues below.

Under a battery of powerful ultraviolet lights, those gowned surgeons operate on a patient whose skull has been opened to reveal the brain. The patient is covered in protective drapes; only her brain is exposed. The spray from an atomiser ensures that the carpet of cortex on the surface of the brain is kept moist. Using platinum electrodes, with sterilised glass handles attached to a stimulator controlling the strength and frequency of the current, one of the surgeons probes and maps out the cortex, placing tiny numbered tags on the regions of the brain identified with particular sensations by the still-conscious patient. At one stage the probe stimulating the cortex elicits a familiar response: slow clonic contractions around the jaw, similar to those the patient had experienced when having seizures.

By specifically identifying the site of the origin of the abnormal electrical activity the surgeons should be able, when excising the scar tissue, to avoid damaging nearby delicate brain matter potentially responsible for vital functions, these areas already having been mapped in the process.

It all seemed in the realm of science fiction to viewers in the 1960s. In the film, Penfield makes the case for brain exploration over space exploration, for the study of the brain's millions of neurones which 'constitute a microcosm that is just as vast as the universe'.

The BBC documentary makers were unashamedly as enthralled as the public by Dr Penfield's demonstrations and particularly by his revelation of one of the most exciting and astonishing offshoots of the Montreal procedure: the discovery in a small number of patients that a mild electrical current applied to the surface of the brain, stimulated by the probes at certain regions, brought about the recall in the patient of a specific memory from his own past.

When Penfield first began operating under the principles that would become the Montreal procedure a patient's response to the electrical stimulation was a good indicator of where the surgeon should make his incision but it could not be relied upon; it could only ever be an approximation. Further confirmation came from X-rays and the primitive use of electroencephalography (then in its infancy). Dr Penfield and his colleagues were consequently very cautious. But though they reported improvements in some patients, it soon became obvious that if the neocortical excisions were fully to control the epilepsy, the surgeons would need to go further and cut deeper – towards the hippocampus. Penfield had shied away from the hippocampus because of its size and beauty, and suspicions of its importance. But, recalled the psychologist Brenda Milner, as more and more patients returned from surgery with their epilepsy still beyond their control, Penfield took the decision that he and his team would need to be bolder; they decided to excise a part of the hippocampus known as the amygdala and additional brain tissue from the medial temporal region.[29]

The risks seemed to be borne out by the successes that followed but there was at least one sobering and unexpected consequence in a small number of people who underwent the temporal lobe operations: an impairment of their memory. A couple of patients (in quick succession) reported severe amnesia. Following surgery, one of the patients, P.B., a civil engineer, could not remember what had happened in his daily life. It angered him and routinely he would berate the staff with the sarcastic comment, 'What have you people done to my memory?'[30]

The memory loss exhibited by these patients mirrored that of the twenty-seven-year-old man known as H.M. who had a long history of minor and major convulsions uncontrolled by medication which prevented him from working. In 1953 H.M. had been oper- ated on by a surgeon in the USA using a much more radical technique for a bilateral resection (i.e. on both sides of the temporal lobes). The front half of both sides of his hippocampus, and the majority of the amygdala, were scooped out – with tragic consequences. H.M., who was later identified as Henry Gustav Molaison, of Hartford, Connecticut, had subsequently been referred to Brenda Milner at the neurological institute in Montreal.

Henry Molaison had suffered disastrous memory impairment. Straight after the operation he could not recognise any member of staff, nor find his way around the hospital. He could not hold on to the memory of any day-to-day event, such as what he'd had for breakfast or even whether he'd eaten breakfast in the first place. Though his early childhood memories were intact, H.M. seemed to be condemned to live in a permanent present, without any recall of events that had only recently passed. Reading the same magazine day after day was of equal interest to him; and the same jigsaw puzzle was just as difficult to complete as the time before, H.M. having gained no benefit from his previous experience of piecing it together. A stranger might have been perplexed to learn that H.M. was incapacitated by these mundane difficulties because his intelligence was not diminished; his understanding and reasoning were intact. But H.M. was a liability to himself. Leaving home in the morning, he would be unable to find his way back because he had no ability to store or recover fresh experiences. Though over the next fifty years Brenda Milner had numerous consultations with him, on each occasion he believed they were meeting for the first time.

H.M.'s tragic loss of short-term memory was to form the bedrock upon which much of medicine's understanding of memory is now based. For example, tests with H.M. enabled scientists to distinguish between conscious and unconscious memory; so that whilst a few minutes after leaving a bicycle shop, H.M. would look perplexedly at the bicycle he was wheeling, having forgotten that he'd just bought it, he could still learn and retain the new motor skills that would enable him later to ride a bicycle.

There were, of course, benefits from his operation. His seizures were much reduced and the surgery had no impact on his cognitive ability. If anything, reported Milner, his general intelligence had improved since the procedure, 'possibly because he is less drowsy than before'. And though H.M. was not plagued by any dark thoughts about his predicament, he still retained the memories of his earlier distressing fits which had compelled him to take the risk of the experimental surgery in the first place.[31]

None of the thousand or more patients who had elected for surgery in the Montreal Institute by the time the BBC filmed there in the 1960s had had such dramatic results as H.M. Ultimately, campaigning and crusading men such as Penfield were galvanised by the potential of this new experimental surgery. It underscored their fundamental belief that 'it becomes evident that human behaviour and mental activity may be more greatly impaired by the positive action of an abnormal area of brain than by the negative effect of its complete absence' i.e. that a 'bad brain is worse than no brain'. It had seemed counter-intuitive that surgeons could remove such large portions of the brain without it having a deleterious effect, but in their pioneering operations Penfield and his colleagues were beginning to realise that whilst damaged areas of brain obviously decreased mental capacity, their removal might 'allow other parts of the brain to recover their normal functions' (in what is now commonly regarded as an example of the brain's plasticity).[32]

Other clinics and institutes around the world have attempted to replicate Montreal's success: '76% of our patients with epilepsy are seizure free, one year after surgery,' trumpets the advert for the Cleveland Clinic, adding, a little smugly, that it is one reason why epileptics from twenty-seven countries made their way to Cleveland last year.

The clinic's potential client base for medical tourism is huge. There are 60 million epileptics on the planet. For more than a third of them, the conventional pharmacological treatments barely keep their conditions in check. Rather, epilepsy seems to be in control of them. Not surprisingly then, there's an active market offering alternatives to drugs.

A quick tour of the Cleveland Clinic's site, however, introduces enough caveats to give even the bravest or most desperate epileptic pause for thought. First there are the operations themselves: surgical removal of the troubled zone of the brain; or vagus nerve stimulation following battery-powered tunnelling to locate the nerve. Then there are the possible side effects of surgery including: vocal cord paralysis, lower facial muscle paresis, cardiac arrest and/ or sudden unexplained death. The statistics suggest that the uptake has not been great.

The National Hospital for Neurology and Neurosurgery in Queen Square seems more conservative and cautious in its approach. I was invited along to the Thursday review meetings where a team of professionals – neurologists, neuropsychiatrists, psychologist, radiologist and social workers – gather to decide on a course of treatment for half a dozen patients, more specifically to determine whether they are suitable candidates for surgery. Their decision/advice, on whether to act or not, is then subsequently relayed to the surgeon. The dynamic is always fascinating. To shuffle from neurologist to neurosurgeon is to move from poetry to prose.

The team assembled; the lights were turned off and the projector was switched on for the display of case histories, notes, electro-encephalograms, video telemetry footage and MRI scans. A sixty-year-old neurology consultant, who clearly retained his boyish enthusiasm for his chosen profession, presided over the meeting. He swivelled constantly and contemplatively in his seat, as if on the swing chair on a porch; the action freed up thought – was an aid to clarity.

Voices emerged out of the darkness. A self-conscious and mono-tone junior member read out the notes projected onto the screen – verbatim, quickly hurrying through, hoping not to make mistakes but making them anyway. He even made perfunctory-sounding the description of the patient whose seizures were like being in a waterfall. The junior doctor was 'good neurosurgeon material' I scribbled in my notes. The radiologist was much more clear and precise. She spoke with the kind of confidence that would not necessarily brook dissent but would be surprised to hear any. The MRI images of the brain expanded and contracted smoothly on screen like TV weather representations of clouds shifting shape with a changing weather pattern.

Mostly the consultant asked questions and the others' jobs were to answer him; except for one of the team from whom he solicited an overall opinion. It seemed odd, given the deference of everyone else, that they were having a dialogue. It was robust but temperate. If they'd been pugilists you might have thought they were shadow boxing or pulling their punches. They differed over one of the patients, a translator, who complained of auras, of 'rising energy from his stomach' and 'night terrors'. The video telemetry showed his strange seizures – bicycling legs kicking off the bed sheets. He was having fifty episodes per night, and seemed a likely candidate for surgery. The consultant was concerned about how much surrounding brain tissue might need to be taken out if they went ahead, and how that might impact on speech/language, especially given that the patient was a translator. The consultant's junior (I assumed a senior registrar) advanced a bolder line, and conceded the case for further investigation, but for the more invasive intra-cranial electrical probes to be inserted deep into the brain and not just on the surface of the cortex.

'Be nice to avoid implantation – as there's dual pathology,' said the consultant.

'It might reduce the odds for success,' answered the senior registrar in a tighter voice than she perhaps intended.

'What would you say is a good success – sixty, seventy per cent?'

'More like fifty, sixty per cent,' said the senior registrar. And then added, 'Please disagree with me.'

At this point I realised my assumption that she was his junior was incorrect: they were both consultants.

'I'm always fearful of these frontal and temporal lobe things,' admitted the male consultant.

'Fearful?'

'Yes. You end up taking out masses of brain.'

The consultants had appeared, to my untrained ear, mutually respectful duellists, but when the lights came up they emerged as more collegiate than competitive – in agreement, notwithstanding that the more cautious of the two seemed better pleased with the result. The case was deferred. It was a good outcome. The discussion marked how the passage of time and an increase in expertise allows for nuance. The team had erred on the side of 'bad brain is *better* than no brain' – for now. Of the six patients none would advance to surgery. Had they been reviewed by Penfield sixty years ago, I suspected all would have been considered suitable candidates.

Even outside surgery, there are many 'non-compliant' epileptics who 'pass' on what the medical profession has to offer. They are un-medicated not by neglect but by choice – the musician, Neil Young, amongst them.

Neil Young has a finely developed cussedness in refusing to be bound by the limits of epilepsy. Seizures are usually a contraindication to driving. But Young was never going to let epilepsy separate him from his prized 1951 Willys Jeepster convertible. As he recalls, the risks were in any event limited, because of the preceding auras: 'I had a warning all my life which I recognised right away – I had a good forty-five seconds to react.'

Among epileptics there is a strong desire to hold on to as many strands as possible of the life they have grown accustomed to prior to their diagnosis. In my brother's case, it seemed to take a very long time for the categorical diagnosis of epilepsy to be made. There were numerous tests before reaching that stage.

Neil Young has been un-medicated for the last twenty years. His disenchantment with the medical treatments on offer dates back to the late sixties when, after a fit on stage, he was admitted to the neuropsychiatric wing of UCLA and underwent a 'barbaric surgical procedure'. Before outlining the details of the operation in his biography, *Waging Heavy Peace*, Young gives the reader fair warning, writing in capitals, 'I DO NOT RECOMMEND THIS TEST.' The procedure was, he remembers, basically a kind of torture: 'A radioactive dye is injected into your blood system and into your nervous system. Then they track it up into your head. [Unfortunately], they usually get some bubbles; so when those go through your brain it's excruciating.'

The doctors didn't learn anything from the test, but decades later, largely free of epileptic episodes, Neil Young is phlegmatic about living with the condition: 'It's a very psychedelic experience to have a seizure. You slip into another world . . . [but] then you reboot. It's just a part of me, part of the landscape.'

Research is still ongoing as to why some people with epilepsy prefer to remain un-medicated. There are myriad reasons. But it is common, for example, for pregnant women to worry about the side effects of medication on their unborn babies. Ultimately it's not a case of compliance over non-compliance; rather it is simply, and sometimes unfathomably, a choice. Surgery is a difficult choice but a choice nonetheless; people after all have elected for surgery.

But ever since the 1930s surgery has historically been a treatment of last resort; a final roll of the dice. For despite the distress and real danger from injury that seizure may cause, despite

Dr Radcliffe's graphic remarks about the invisible executioner's bowstring, death from a direct attack is rare.

At about three o'clock in the morning yet again there was a knock on the front door. I opened it and was confronted by the same policeman who'd knocked a month earlier. This time he did not say my name; but gestured, more wearily than before, towards the police car. Inside was the proof that I, as the responsible adult, had reneged on an unspoken promise. The car door squeaked open.

'At least he has his shoes,' I said.

The policeman's jaw moved back and forth as if he was trying to click it into place.

'The shoes, remember?' I said.

The policeman did not return my smile.

Persona

I never used the words 'seizure' or 'fit' in my brother's presence. Often Christopher would have an epileptic attack without warning and on regaining full consciousness he'd be dismayed to find himself on the floor or on a hospital trolley. We'd both grown tired of the 'you've had a visitor' gag. Now I'd lean over and explain that for a while there, he was 'not in Kansas any more'. It was our new private joke; a shorthand that needed no elaboration. I like to think that in the no-time of the paroxysm and its immediate aftermath Christopher had been astral travelling or had passed through a wonderland – though he had no memory of it.

It wasn't always possible to sustain that tone or that mischievous lightness of being as the grand mal epilepsy raged out of control. The late 1990s were the worst years of attrition when Christopher was pounded with large-scale explosive attacks every few weeks, often dangerously outside when walking on the pavement; and each time it seemed that a bit more of him was chipped away. His mood darkened yet he still refused fully to accept the medication.

After one particularly bruising attack when he slammed into the road on his thirty-first birthday (smashing his glasses that cut into his temple, splitting his lip and lacerating his cheeks on the grit of the tarmac), Christopher eventually opened his eyes and simply said, 'Bagpipes!' Later on he elaborated that, should he die during a seizure, he wanted to have bagpipes played at his funeral. He insisted that I make the pledge. I made a point of not answering him. But after each subsequent fit, Christopher would say the same thing again about bagpipes. And then he started mentioning it in the honeymoon period between fits (interictally as the medics say), randomly, when we were out driving or walking or at the end of viewing a film in the cinema. It went on like this for months. But then suddenly he stopped. Even though it was obvious the sentiment had not left him, bagpipes were never mentioned again.

Living with a chronic condition inevitably has an impact on your character and outlook, but along with Christopher I had scoffed at the notion that epilepsy might affect his temperament. Yet with each fit, there seemed to be subtle shifts in his personality. Christopher appeared to lose something of the innocent persona that charmed everybody, and had begun to turn, to migrate, ever more inwards. He came to live with us (me, my wife and children) at the start of the new millennium and we were struck by his strange, Zen-like stillness. We'd leave him alone in the house in the morning and return in the afternoon or evening to find him uncannily sitting in the same chair, perfectly still. That shutting down I surmised was willed but might it in some way have been the product of the pathology of his epilepsy?

By the year 2000 people with epilepsy no longer had to put up with the primitive and outdated idea of the 'epileptic personality'. Nineteenth-century writing, for example, had been awash with suggestions of behavioural disorders associated with epilepsy: hysteria, epileptic insanity, epileptic mania. The dangerous, criminal epileptic depicted as a kind of Jekyll and Hyde capable of murder in the fog of confusion following a seizure was as likely to be found in medical textbooks as he was in works of fiction. As late as the 1940s the Swedish neurologist, Sjorbing, no doubt thought he was writing sympathetically when he concluded, 'A mental change of a specific nature takes place in individuals suffering from epileptic seizures. They become torpid and circumstantial, sticky and adhesive, effectively tense, and suffer from explosive outbursts of rage, anxiety, etc.'[1]

But medicine, science and society evolved with the realisation that such prejudicial thinking was a libel on all people with epilepsy, and had largely contributed to the stigma attached to the condition. The uncoupling of epilepsy from mental ill health further distanced any association of epilepsy with personality disorders. Nonetheless, in the 1950s neurologists began recording cases of people with temporal lobe epilepsy (TLE) who were coming into clinics complaining of disturbing changes in their personalities. Evidently, these specialists struggled to write about what they were witnessing without suggesting the kind of behavioural disorder more commonly associated with psychiatric patients. This was dramatically illustrated by researchers in 1954 at the Maudsley Hospital in London, reporting on the unusual case of a man for whom looking at a safety pin could trigger both sexual arousal and an epileptic seizure.[2]

Since childhood, the thirty-eight-year-old patient had enjoyed what he called 'thought satisfaction' when staring at a safety pin. The habit continued into marriage when, during sexual intercourse, he would imagine the pin. This arousal which culminated in an orgasm was followed by a 'blank period' – a petit mal preceded by *la petite mort*. His wife had been unaware of the ritual, but then, unexpectedly, she'd caught sight of him (outside of intimacy), staring at a pin for a minute; he appeared glassy-eyed, began to hum and suck in his lips and finally stood stock-still for a minute or two before recovering. The same thing happened several other times, until after a while his wife noted another worrying trend: her husband started dressing himself in her clothes, and wearing them not just at home but in public as well. What did it all mean? The researchers were unsure. They could only speculate because 'the mechanism whereby the gratification of the fetish-need either became attached to the mechanism for the onset of the epileptic seizure or became the immediate precipitant thereof must, of course, remain obscure'.[3]

The most relevant question, arguably, was not which came first, the fetishistic arousal or the epileptic seizure, but how the regions of the brain were connected, so that stimulation in one focus could elicit seizure-like *and* emotional responses. Along with his history an EEG established the diagnosis of temporal lobe epilepsy (TLE) and he subsequently underwent brain surgery (a temporal lobectomy). The seizures ceased immediately as did the fetishistic response: the patient was no longer aroused by the sight of a safety pin.

By the time the Harvard neurologist Norman Geschwind entered into the debate in the 1970s it was clear that there was growing evidence and numbers of patients to support the claim that, however counter-intuitive it seemed, there might be an organic basis to the personality changes in some patients with TLE. Characteristically the lesions producing the epilepsy are on the inner surface of the temporal lobe in structures with pathways to those parts of the brain involved in emotional behaviour. Geschwind argued that the reaction to the epileptic stimulus is modified as it travels through the limbic system to the brain's emotional centres.[4] The safety-pin man was rare but not unique. In 1980 Geschwind reported on the case of a woman referred for evaluation because of 'exhibitionism'. The exhibitionism had a sexual flavour. The woman confessed that she was aroused in church, and that in particular she had experienced orgasms brought on by vaginal tingling while focusing on the crucifix. Treatment with Carbamazepine had helped to curb her hyper-sexuality but her provocative dressing continued as did her demands for frequent sexual intercourse from her husband.

Such cases led Geschwind to conceive of a cluster of behavioural change symptoms which he believed were firmly associated with temporal lobe epilepsy. The symptoms of this so-called Geschwind's syndrome described a phenomenon that occurred interictally, between seizures. They included a propensity towards becoming aggressive over trivial matters. Geschwind cited numerous examples of patients' exaggerated concerns over morality and fairness. A patient might, for example, vehemently object to being told to put out his cigarette until it could be shown that no one else in the entire hospital was allowed to smoke. Hyper-religiosity and an obsession with cosmic concerns also featured prominently, including people with religious conversions and ecstatic auras. There were striking changes in sexual behaviour, most commonly in a loss of sexual interest or sexual reorientation. And some patients also showed a marked tendency towards over-explication, conveyed by excessive writing, which was occasionally underlined and highlighted to stress importance. In one instance Geschwind's fellow researcher employed a court stenographer for a patient whose dictation ran to more than twenty hours.

Establishing a clear and consistent diagnostic framework, though, proved elusive. The picture was often confusing; especially in patients where there appeared to be an overlap between neurological and psychiatric symptoms. The troubles of Philip K. Dick were a case in point.

20 February 1974 did not begin well for the science-fiction writer, Philip K. Dick. Partial relief from an impacted wisdom tooth came courtesy of a pair of dentist's pliers and a dose of sodium pentothal. But Dick needed topping up with further anaesthesia. Later that evening, the pharmacist's delivery girl arrived at

his home with a welcome bottle of Darvon tablets. But what she wore round her neck proved a bigger distraction than the drugs.

Not immediately but soon after, the medallion – a golden fish (an ancient Christian symbol) – started to emit a dazzling ray of pink light. Philip K. Dick later claimed he experienced the most wondrous epiphany; that he and the delivery girl were early Christians, in flight from Roman persecution. They couldn't speak directly about it but the code was clear. Dick understood that he wasn't having a flashback to Rome in AD 70, but that it *was* AD 70. The Roman Empire had yet to come to an end and 1974 was yet to happen. His *previous* sensory state, prior to the delivery girl's arrival, was the illusion.

Dick's description was not unlike the accounts of double-consciousness (of being in the present and past at the same time) that some sufferers of partial complex seizures have expressed, and as was noted by Gowers and Hughlings Jackson in the nineteenth century. It didn't stop there. In that moment, claimed the writer, the total recall of human knowledge was revealed to him. And there was more. In the days and nights that followed Dick wrote that he was exposed to the kind of psychedelic visions and phantasmagorical illuminations usually only found on the CVs of mystics (or in the case notes of partial epileptics). They included 'hundreds of thousands of absolutely terrific modern art pictures as good as any ever exhibited; a red and gold plasmatic entity; and a radio that played without being turned on or plugged into the socket.'

What is the rational explanation for that night? Much of Philip K. Dick's writing career to date seemed to have been an audition for 20 February 1974. In the 1950s and 1960s, submerged in writing, fuelled by a chemical cocktail of drugs, and barely coming up for air, he produced more than thirty novels. It has been argued that Dick, the eccentric science-fiction writer whose novel *Do Androids*

Dream of Electric Sheep? would later be transformed into the movie *Blade Runner*, might have experienced transient ischaemic attacks or a temporary stroke on that night, or that his neurochemistry went awry following a prodigious intake of amphetamines (for which he was renowned).

But some neurologists have postulated that Philip K. Dick's symptoms bore a closer resemblance to someone suffering from Geschwind's personality syndrome. He certainly ticked many of the relevant boxes, including hyper-religiosity, fits of remembrance, being overly concerned with details but struggling to get to the point, and especially hypergraphia (excessive writing). Notwithstanding that throughout his writing career his output had been prodigious, Dick turned up the writing dial way past eleven.

Whether from the result of temporal lobe epilepsy or not, Dick's report of the visual phenomena of 20 February corresponds with accounts of people who have experienced hallucinations that were not triggered by an external stimulus: 'the original display of dazzling graphics which I saw . . . were characterised by their balance, not what shapes they contained. They were, like much of Kandinsky's abstract art, modern aesthetic elaborations, in colour, of the ancient a priori geometric forms conceived by the Greeks. They were permutations of the Golden Rectangle.'[5]

Philip K. Dick's initial intrigue developed into an obsession. Over the next eight years he assembled a battery of scholarly books and encyclopaedias – stacked high on his desk and spread out to cover every inch of floor space in his study – in an attempt to explain to himself and to the future reader what had happened in the aftermath of the epiphany and what it meant. The obsession ran high in his veins and flowed through his arms onto paper, writing through the night, sometimes completing dozens of pages of closely lined text in one sitting. By the end of Dick's life,

Exegesis, his hypergraphia on the ramifications of the 'golden fish' incident, ran to more than 8,000 pages.

The difficulty of faithfully rendering the experience is evident in those pages. There are extraordinarily lucid intervals, ruminations on metaphysics and mysticism and florid megalomaniacal moments of self-indulgence. In part this is explained by the absence of an editor at his elbow but more so by the fevered hypergraphia which grew and grew, informed by the detritus of auditory and visual hallucinations.

Exegesis was his last work; and the first extract of it (a mere 950 pages) was posthumously published in 2011 – a partial recall of the literary re-enactment of the night he encoded '2-3-74' (a reference to the hypnagogic events of the second and third months of 1974). Ultimately, it is an investigation of its own enquiry, spanning years and spinning ideas like plates on a juggler's stick.

The jury is still out on this last defining phase of the science-fiction writer's life; the popular ambivalence is captured by Adam Gopnik's description of *Valis*, another of Dick's novels inspired by the post-dental extraction, as 'a work of cosmic explanation in which lightning bolts of brilliance flash over salty oceans of insanity'.[6]

But more than a literary achievement, Philip K. Dick's *Exegesis* acts as a gateway to his psychological make-up. The trauma, whatever its origins, was an insult to the brain, and provided a door to his transcendence. Dick took a glimpse through that portal and heroically tried to explain it to himself and to his future readers. He had pursued more prosaic meanings through the prism of contemporary medicine but nothing seemed to fit. Several times in *Exegesis* he ponders whether he is simply schizophrenic. After all, one of his provocative aphorisms or aphoristic provocations was that 'the schizophrenic is the leap ahead that failed.'[7] But Dick recalled that a psychiatrist once told him, 'I could not be diagnosed due to the unusual life I had led. Since I saw him I have led an even more unusual life and therefore I suppose diagnosis is even more difficult now.'[8]

Perhaps Dick could not be diagnosed because the language of psychiatry, the lexicon of that discipline, did not fit what he was going through. All too often it has been assumed that psychiatry offers the best model to describe some of the behaviours and personality changes in temporal lobe epilepsy, but maybe these behaviours only have the appearance of similarity, and that something altogether different is going on in the brain. Geschwind stressed this when he spoke of personality *change* rather than personality *disorder*. A change in a patient's religious outlook, a conversion, should no more worry the physician, he argued, than if his patient had switched allegiance from one political party (Democrat) to the other (Republican). 'It is not a disorder if it is not disabling to the patient or to those around him.'[9]

The debate about neurological conditions vs. psychiatric illness has surfaced again in recent years with the focus on misdiagnosis. As late as 1988, a third of patients with temporal lobe epilepsy who were treated at the Beth Israel Hospital in Boston were first misdiagnosed with a psychiatric disorder. A number of mentally ill patients would willingly trade their psychiatric diagnosis for an epileptic one. In the hierarchy of stigmas, mental ill health still tops any neurological condition. People such as Philip K. Dick, Dostoevsky and Van Gogh show us just how porous the borders are between neurological and psychological complaints.

There are many neurologists who doubt the organic roots of Geschwind's syndrome, suggesting rather that so-called personality alterations occur not because of physiological or neurological changes but are more likely to be the result of the psychological and social stresses that all epilepsy sufferers experience.

Even if we reject the notion of the epileptic personality it does not preclude the possibility, for example, of bipolar and epileptic characteristics residing in an individual and for both to impact on that individual's creativity.

The neurologist Norman Geschwind thought that Dostoevsky's epilepsy exemplified many of the personality characteristics of his syndrome: 'tremendous concern about moral details, many of them small details, extremely pedantic, he was angrily impulsive . . . an impossible person to live with in every way, and extremely aggressive, even toward people who had befriended him'. Geschwind introduces Dostoevsky as an anomaly whose hypergraphia, like Philip K. Dick's, but unlike the majority of such cases, is of high literary merit. Other neurologists and neuropsychologists, such as Paul Spiers, have gone even further in making the questionable and speculative link between the syndrome and creative writing.

A poet and TLE patient of Spiers used to complain that 'when her seizures are under control, the muse leaves her'.[10] Might Dostoevsky have written as much as he did because of the behavioural changes wrought by his epilepsy? Geschwind believed so but he cautioned that: 'Epilepsy may help to account for the content, but it cannot explain genius.' There can be little doubt, though, that Dostoevsky's epilepsy was hugely impactful on his writing life and philosophy: 'The principal question I will deal with in every part of my novel is the one about which I have suffered all my life, consciously or unconsciously,' he wrote, 'the problem of God's existence.'[11]

It's clear from his diaries and the accounts of his wife and friends that Dostoevsky transposed much of his own experience of epilepsy into his novels and stories, and on some occasions the biographical and fictional accounts are almost interchangeable; so that Prince Myshkin, the protagonist of *The Idiot*, appears to be channelling the writer.

In a 1960s lecture devoted to an analysis of Dostoevsky's epilepsy, the neurologist Théophile Alajouanine, having fastidiously noted every reference to epilepsy in Dostoevsky's work, concluded, 'It would be naive to consider that Dostoevsky's epilepsy is the essential origin of his genius, but it was surely an exceptional experience which had driven him towards manifesting his original vision. In point of fact, epilepsy had created in the person of Dostoevsky a "double man": a rationalist and a mystic; each having the better of the other according to the moment; more and more the mystical one seems to have prevailed.'[12]

Towards the end of his book *Exegesis*, Philip K. Dick worries, not for the first time, about the value of his obsession. His exegesis he confesses 'is both a delusion in which I am trapped and, in addition, a delusion *I am creating for others*'.[13]

But the study and understanding of TLE may lead to a better comprehension and treatment of mental ill heath such as schizophrenia. Research that has been able to identify the location of the lesions responsible for behavioural changes in epilepsy and to advance credible theories as to the mechanisms involved, holds out hope for illuminating the opaque mechanisms and sources in psychiatric illness whose manifestations in behavioural change appear close to, or overlap with, TLE. We now know for instance that traffic between epilepsy and depression leads both ways – people with epilepsy are as much predisposed towards depression as those with depression are predisposed to epilepsy.[14] The hope is that in the future we will find out why that is so.

At some stage in their lives everyone who has been diagnosed with epilepsy will be presented with the list: those notable people, past and present, who have also been diagnosed with the condition. The crowd-sourced encyclopaedia, Wikipedia, lists more than 100 people from Vladimir Ilyich Lenin to Harriet Tubman – with various caveats and qualifications, especially as retrospective diagnoses for historical figures are near impossible to substantiate.

The artist Vincent Van Gogh doesn't make the cut on the Wikipedia list; he is relegated to the also-rans list of notables with 'similar conditions' to epilepsy. But for many neurologists Van Gogh's story is a compelling and unambiguous account of a man whose strange changes in behaviour were the result of temporal lobe epilepsy, and offer further evidence of Geschwind's syndrome.

Van Gogh's medical history also highlights the ongoing debate about the value of individual case reports over large-scale group studies. Peer-reviewed journals consider double-blinded, randomised controlled studies a necessary benchmark, if not the gold standard, for advancing medicine. But Geschwind and like-minded scientists have worried about the notion that 'people measure what can be measured', that is, what the thinker thinks, the prover proves. This applies to some large-scale studies in which, although statistical comparisons between large groups appear to yield something significant, they are later found to have no real biological or clinical meaning; and that medicine fails to reap the lessons, learnt by figures such as Hughlings Jackson and Gowers, about the insights gleaned from the concentrated focus on an individual case.[15]

There are numerous retrospective explanations for Van Gogh's bizarre behaviour which famously culminated in him cutting off part of his ear before his eventual suicide in 1890. Having spied a sprig of foxglove in Van Gogh's portrait of his therapist, Dr Gachet, one forensic sleuth leapt to the diagnosis of digitalis poisoning which he assumed explained the 'high yellow tone' in several paintings. Excessive consumption of absinthe as a probable cause for Van Gogh's seizures has divided experts. But the most rancorous arguments centre on the suggested diagnosis of epilepsy – giving rise to extraordinarily self-serving and petulant academic spats. Whilst many concede that Vincent Van Gogh's case presents one of the best examples of Geschwind syndrome, the notion that the artist suffered from epilepsy sticks in their craw. As one researcher put it, 'If there is no clear temporal lobe epilepsy, then the syndrome is an orphan without a parent condition.'[16] No reputation is spared in identifying those guilty of the folly of misdiagnosis, not even the original doctor or the patient himself.

Yet Van Gogh's epilepsy is spelt out in his correspondence with his brother Theo. The neurologist Fabienne Picard is amongst those who think that the publications of the letters 'make the diagnosis of epilepsy indisputable'. The transcript of the doctor's notes on Van Gogh's admission to the St Remy Mental Home on 9 May 1889 records that the artist had 'suffered an attack of acute mania with visual and auditory hallucinations that led him to mutilate himself by cutting off his ear . . . Based on all the above, I consider that Mr. van Gogh is subject to attacks of epilepsy, separated by long intervals.'[17]

Lengthy but lucid letters from Vincent to his brother came thick and fast in the late 1880s – a period in which he also produced hundreds of paintings and drawings. The letters chart how precarious and unpredictable life could be for a sufferer of epilepsy and its impact on his mental health. A few months later, on 5 October, Van Gogh appeared particularly anxious about the consequences of having any subsequent fit in public. He wrote to his brother that he was keen to become acquainted with the doctor in the next town to which he intended to travel, 'so that in the event of a crisis, one doesn't fall into the hands of the police and isn't forcibly carried off into any asylum'.

The last word has yet to be expressed on that which ailed Van Gogh's mind. The same is true for the value and inspiration of his paintings. Decades of poring over his work by amateurs and professionals – art historians, critics, psychologists and neurologists, all attempting to tease out the relation of his art to his mind – has reduced Van Gogh to the cliché of the crazy, starving artist genius whose work (the heaving, throbbing, radiating paintings and violent, swirling drawings) is an index of his madness.

But one value of Van Gogh to the story of epilepsy is the certainty that though the condition is challenging (and even more so when the person with epilepsy is in the grip of Geschwind's syndrome), it need not be disabling. Nevertheless, people such as my brother would take little comfort from the oft-repeated assertion, 'Look at Van Gogh, look at Caesar, look at Harriet Tubman – they still got on with their lives.'

The eminent and mischievous behavioural neurologist V. S. Ramachandran believes that Van Gogh's epilepsy may have given him an advantage. In his reflections on 'The Science of Art', Ramachandran proposes a theory:

> Van Gogh's epileptic seizures in his temporal lobes may have actually strengthened neural connections between his visual object and face area and the amygdala, nucleus accumbens and other brain regions involved in gauging the emotional significance of what's being viewed. Such a heightened attention and emotional response to visual images may have made him a more accomplished artist – his seizures enabling him to 'attend' to certain critical dimensions more than you or I.[18]

It is impossible to accurately trace the line between Van Gogh's art and his mental condition. But it *is* indisputable that Van Gogh's final fecund years were a riot of fevered output both in his hypergraphia and his art. Hundreds of letters, more than a thousand drawings and almost as many paintings survived. His artist's incontinence was a mark of his urgency to get down that which was imperative for him to express. Epilepsy accelerated the process.

*

In 2007, after years of sleepwalking through piecemeal and short-term jobs, Christopher finally woke up. He had a calling. He was going to be a film-maker. He assembled cameras, editing software and an array of film equipment. I contributed with a loan. He was, he said, going to make a British version of *Koyaanisqatsi*. But he would start by making short films to reveal what was going on inside his epileptic mind. One day he called me over to his flat to view a rough cut of the first film. I was keen to see how my investment had paid off. It was a bright afternoon. We drew the curtains to shut out the light, and sat in front of his laptop. The screen was black, with an occasional flicker of what looked like static.

'I think you need to reboot the computer,' I said.

'Oh, man,' said Christopher. 'Can't you see? I expected you, of all people, to see.'

'See what?'

'This is it. It's running. The film.'

'You're having a laugh,' I chortled, and wished I hadn't. Christopher did not laugh along with me.

'This is not a joke, joke t'ing, you know, bredren,' said Christopher sharply. 'This isn't something else. This is it.'

'This is the film?' I asked. 'But it's just a blank screen.'

'Take a closer look.'

I sat and stared, and attempted to drain my face of the last vestige of scepticism. I did not succeed. Christopher was upset but I was blind to what he could see. I thought of that film when I put on a pair of virtual-reality goggles seven years later. I was handed them by J, the young woman who had developed epilepsy following her brain surgery after she was mugged. Before her assault J had embarked on a career in the theatre; and now she had devised an individual theatre show based on one of her epileptic seizures that had occurred on a train journey that went awry. She hoped, through the use of a virtual-reality headset, to capture for an audience that awful sickening moment when the seizure begins and you collapse down the Alice-in-Wonderland hole of surreality.

'I had a seizure when I was in Oxford, and I got a train to go home and I had another really bad seizure and woke up in Slough. And I was trying to work out how I could put other people into my shoes. I'm really interested in how far I can push an audience and how close I can get to them having this experience.'

I put on J's goggles and headphones. The show began. Within a few seconds I appeared to be on a fast-moving train, speeding through the countryside. Somewhere in the distance were the conductor's voice and other passengers, coming in and out like a radio being tuned. Suddenly the train started to shake violently from side to side; there was a terrifying, sharp screeching of the train's brakes apparently being slammed on; and then the screen went black.

It helped, said J, that the virtual-reality technology was still primitive. The goggles were at the point in their development at which they made people sick when wearing them; travel sick. 'It was a bit mean – but I know that it might take them a bit closer to what it's like to have a seizure.'

Epilepsy is so pervasive that it should not be a surprise that an artist's creativity is affected by it. Resistance is impossible, but also necessary. 'I don't have epilepsy,' says the writer M. 'I am epileptic.' It's an important distinction. M admits that it took him as many years to accept it: 'To accept that this is it, that it's never going to end, that it's always going to be a problem.' There is no respite; no divorce or possible settlement. For years M never considered writing about his epilepsy – taking the view that the person with epilepsy is an unreliable witness to his/her seizures. 'We aren't around at the critical moment and have no memory of it . . . Memory is also the first condition of story. Without it, nothing makes sense. The epileptic story is redacted. We start the story and find it has [a gap] in it.'

Epilepsy may not give the sufferer a personality but it casts that person as a character in its story. But the story of epilepsy has been a slow and torturous journey towards acceptance. Along the way, rejection and persecution have been the dominant default positions. A snapshot across the ages, even for those whose public standing gives them greater leverage, makes for unsettling reading.

Though the roll call of epileptics through history is long and impressive, few, I imagine, would have been happy to see themselves inducted into an epileptics' hall of fame. For many, rather than a badge of honour, epilepsy was an emblem of guilt and shame. Would they want to be part of such a club? Nonetheless, over the centuries, so many exceptional people have turned out to be epileptic that the condition was once thought of as a mark of intelligence.[19]

In the last decade this has led researchers in Australia to investigate the links between epilepsy and creativity. More than sixty artists with epilepsy volunteered in the University of Melbourne study 'Sparks of Creativity' to investigate the hypothesis that 'temporolimbic epilepsy . . . leads to altered functioning and hyper stimulation of areas of the brain that control the functions that most influence the creative process'.

The lead researcher is the artist Jim Chambliss who was knocked unconscious in a car accident in 1986 and subsequently developed epilepsy. Chambliss's thesis rests on the concept of 'intrinsic perceptions' (spontaneously and independently derived from the brain in simple or complex hallucinations). Intrinsic perceptions occur, he believes, when sensory experience in people with focal epilepsy 'is so altered by the neurological processes impacted by the misfiring of electrical impulses that what would be commonly perceived or understood as "real" takes on surreal or dreamlike qualities'.

Drawing on Colin Martindale's *Biological Theory of Creativity*, the researcher proposes that intrinsic perceptions can occur in the chaotic state of focal epileptic discharge between one seizure and the next, when 'simultaneous activation of nodes in the brain is more free-flowing'. And if the artist is conscious and fortunate enough to remember and incorporate these perceptions into their art, then Chambliss believes their 'original and novel nature makes the artistic expression inherently more likely to be creative'.

In his theory the timing is crucial as it relies on the potentiality of epileptic discharges between seizures that the artist may not be aware of. At this time, 'when the transient phenomena of epilepsy are more intense', the artists in the study reported such a compulsion to produce art that it might leave them overwrought and on the threshold of collapse.

They ended up creating art, says Chambliss, 'that is dreamlike, surreal or extraordinarily imaginative'. The findings (which are themselves extraordinary) have not been reproduced elsewhere. Another recent paper on epilepsy and art concluded that if there was a common theme among its surveyed artists it was of 'unwanted psychological harm of some seizures provoking dark, frustrated imagery'.[20]

Having flirted with the idea of an artist's epilepsy actually producing the art, Chambliss draws back from making that assertion in his conclusion. He points out not unreasonably (or unsurprisingly) the likelihood of free will and skill being the final arbiter in artistic production whether the artist has epilepsy or not. I would add luck and industry into the mix.

From the letters between Vincent Van Gogh and his brother Theo it is clear that unpredictability and fear of his epilepsy kept

Vincent on amber alert. 'I am not strictly speaking mad, for my mind is absolutely normal in the intervals . . . but during the attacks it is terrible – and then I lose consciousness of everything.' It was why Van Gogh prized his lucid moments. His epilepsy gave him a sense of urgency and spurred on his art: 'It drives me to work and to seriousness, as a coal-miner who is always in danger makes haste in what he does.'[21]

Grand Mal

There was no history of epilepsy in our family. Why Christopher developed it is a mystery: 'God for tell,' as my mother would say. But if God knew, he wasn't telling. Many forms of epilepsy are idiopathic: science has yet to discover what causes it in the majority of cases, and why some individuals are predisposed towards it. There is no cure for epilepsy; treatment of the condition is symptomatic. But in a third of patients the anti-epileptic medication is not effective. Any pharmacological advance is hampered by the ignorance of the profession. Neuroscientists do not yet understand what's going on pathologically at a molecular level. The best hope for illumination seems to lie in discovering genetic variations that might account for increased susceptibility to epilepsy.

Statistically it is known that genetics somehow plays a part. You are four times more at risk (than the general population) of developing epilepsy if you have a sibling or parent with the disorder. But apart from very rare types of epilepsy, with multiple members of a family suffering from the condition over several generations, it hasn't been possible to identify the obvious genetic mutations associated with the disease. For the major, common forms of epilepsy, the genetic cause may be the result of combinations of gene mutations. Since 2007, the Epilepsy Phenome/Genome Project has been gathering critical 'phenotype' data on people with epilepsy as a first step to matching the data to the whole genome of those individuals. In doing so, researchers hope to work out the degree to which combination of mutations in multiple genes might determine a person's susceptibility to seizures.

The researchers have collected blood samples and the clinical details of more than 4,000 patients with epilepsy and their family members; and they have already made preliminary findings in two of the more common types of epilepsy (infantile spasms and Lennox-Gastaut syndrome) believed to arise from 'de novo' mutations (a new variation in a gene that appears for the first time in a family) at or during birth.[1] By also analysing the DNA of parents of children with the condition, but who are free of epilepsy themselves, the researchers were able to isolate the genetic mutations. Nine of these de novo mutations were discovered on specific genes, four of which had never previously been associated with epilepsy.

Futuristic and fanciful not so long ago, each year brings the promise of gene therapy a little nearer, with the tantalising prospect of personalised medicine targeted to the individual based on such information revealed from their genetic make-up. But what if there'd been a marker for epilepsy before the births of the people with epilepsy explored in this book?

Antiquity does not offer much comfort. A baby suspected of epilepsy in ancient Sparta, for example, was washed in wine to see whether he convulsed. If the council of elders judged him unfit, the baby would be taken to Apothetae, a pit near Mount Taygetus, discarded and left to die.

If there'd been an identifiable gene for epilepsy and their parents were presented with the evidence, how many foetal epileptics would have made it even beyond the first trimester? Perhaps we might be surprised by the results. Amongst people with disabilities and their families there is a rigorous debate over ownership of their conditions – at a basic level this focuses on the wisdom or not of embracing or taking possession of names that were previously deemed offensive: dwarf, cripple, etc.

The writer M seems to have taken up this position with his insistence that he is not someone with epilepsy; he is epileptic: 'I am the autonomous agent but I don't have complete agency. Whether any of us does is another thing,' says M. 'But in the case of people with epilepsy their agency, their "I", is sabotaged or compromised by something that they cannot get rid of. I don't want to privilege epilepsy over another condition there is no cure for, but I know that the epilepsy is a determining factor. It constrains my abilities and directs me in a number of ways that I simply can't control, and occasionally the epilepsy will take control of me, or would if I didn't take my medication. But the consequences of the treatment and the side effects of the treatment are altering anyway. They alter you, so whichever way you look at it, you can't come off the treatment and you can't come off the epilepsy.'

Towards the end of our conversation, M turned to me and asked me a startling question, one that I had never considered: 'Would you ever have liked to have been epileptic like your brother?'

I am stunned by the simplicity of the question, and then over-come by its magnitude, by its profundity. What M is really asking is, would I have liked to have experienced what Christopher went through in order to gain some better understanding of it? I spool back through the years, dropping through the trapdoor of time, through the lift shaft of vertiginous memories of the myriad occa-sions I saw my brother have seizures, and was numbed by the utter helplessness of it: there was nothing that could be done other than to try to ensure he didn't further injure himself and to make him comfortable until the fit passed. I repeat M's question out loud. It doesn't make it any easier. I cannot answer. To answer truthfully 'no' would be to consign my brother to a life I know I could not bear – at least not in the way he lived it.[2]

There might be some benefit from experiencing a day in the life of a person with epilepsy. But a day doesn't scale to a life. Epilepsy is not like a coat you can put on or take off.

There was always a moment as the phone rang in the early hours of the morning when my heart was flooded with dread. It could only mean one thing: Christopher had had another fit. The attacks were still random but their effect on him seemed incrementally deleterious; the cuts and gashes deeper and the bruises longer lasting.

On 4 August 2008, the phone rang at about 5 a.m. But even after years of expectancy, of living on the threshold of amber alert, there was always a possibility of a false alarm. I took a deep diver's breath and answered. It was my sister Sonia on the line. Christopher was at her flat, five minutes from where I lived. He was unwell. Could I come over?

'Has he had another turn?' I asked.

'Just come,' she said.

I hurried to my car and drove the short distance to her flat but I could not find anywhere to park on the street. All of the places outside the flat were taken by three ambulances; they were parked with their engines off but with their warning lights ominously, silently flashing.

My mother sat on a low wall outside the flat, talking to herself and to her Lord. In between she leaned over and straightened again, trying and failing to take in air; she couldn't breathe; all the while she made a strange unearthly pitiful sound; her arms flapped uncontrollably. I had never witnessed her in such distress. Throughout our childhood, and into our adulthood, she had always been a fiercely protective guardian, shielding us from the vagaries of the outside world. But she sat there now like a broken sentry lamenting that the barricade had been breached. I did not stop to comfort my mother. Her anguish propelled me towards the open front door. My sister made way, pointing towards the kitchen.

Inside, Christopher lay dying on the kitchen floor. His giant frame filled the room. Either side of him two paramedics worked at massaging his heart back to life.

A third man in a green jumpsuit, who was already packing away some of the equipment, addressed me in a hushed conspiratorial voice. 'Your brother's been under fifteen minutes now. There's not much more we can do. After fifteen minutes . . . It's always upsetting for the team. But I think we're going to have to stop. OK?'

'I'd like to try,' I said. 'I know how.'

The paramedics moved out of the way and I knelt beside my brother and tried to depress his chest. There was no 'give' in his torso. It seemed almost wooden. I was grateful that his eyes were already closed.

I had often pondered the connection between sleep and epilepsy. In his treatise *On Sleep and Waking*, reflecting on the relationship between the two, Aristotle drew the parallel: 'Sleep is like epilepsy, and, in a sense, actually is a seizure of this sort. Accordingly, the beginning of this malady takes place with many during sleep, and their subsequent habitual seizures occur in sleep, not in waking hours.'

Watching Christopher in the throes of an epileptic seizure was always disturbing and distressing. But in the mini drama of the fit, there was always one thing that I looked forward to: the magical moment when Christopher was roused from his slumber after the attack and woke up. In the years since I witnessed my first seizure as a medical student, there had been numerous occasions to reflect on the pertinence of that experience; when watching over my brother in the aftermath of a seizure I would implore him, as I did now, to wake up, to just awake.

After a few minutes of my pointless attempt at cardiac massage, I stood and gestured to the paramedics, surrendering Christopher to them. They had kept their distance respectfully, but now, almost relieved it seemed, they began to unwrap and unzip the black body-bag.

My sister had been hovering on the other side of the kitchen door, and as I passed through she asked, 'Is he all right? Is Chris OK now?'

'No, Sonia,' I said. 'He's gone. He's gone.'

He was gone, 'gone to foreign', as Jamaicans say. Yet in the hours after Christopher's death my mother and sister reported, separately and together, moments when they had felt his presence. I was summoned in the early evening and ushered into the bedroom where Christopher had spent his last night, and beckoned to look at the brickwork around the fireplace. Did I not see, as they did, the outline of Christopher rendered in the rugged bricks?

There was an inevitability about Christopher's death; and yet when it came it had been sudden and unexpected. He was thirty-nine. Having waved on the paramedics to do their work, almost immediately after they'd taken his body away in the ambulance, I regretted surrendering him so meekly. I phoned the authorities for them to return Christopher to us but they would not. He was in the system now and already being processed for an autopsy; and it was then that I heard for the first time the expression, SUDEP, sudden unexpected death in epilepsy – which would also be the coroner's verdict as to cause of death. Christopher had no history of heart problems; he was fit, and yet during his last seizure he had suffered a massive heart attack.

Our family ignorance in part related to the fact that Christopher would not discuss his condition. Over a century ago doctors had identified SUDEP, though the term had not yet been coined. In his 1904 book on treatment, William Spratling described the risk from epilepsy that 'destroys life suddenly and without warning through a single, brief attack and does so in from 3 to 4% of all who suffer from it.'[3]

SUDEP is the leading cause of death in people whose epilepsy is uncontrolled. In the UK a thousand people a year die from epilepsy-related causes, and more than half of them as a consequence of SUDEP. 'A few hundred people may not sound like a lot,' reflects the neurologist, Professor Ley Sander, 'but the majority of these people are young and in the prime of their lives.' There have been studies to clarify who might be at risk; but confirmation is still some way off. In the meantime, doctors tread a fine line in determining when and how to educate patients and their friends and relatives about the risks without unnecessarily scaring them into cranking up from amber to red the levels of uncertainty of life lived on alert.

It's unlikely that we'd have been any more vigilant had we known that Christopher was vulnerable to SUDEP. To begin to think otherwise, as I did, was to begin to be undermined by the false memories of my past inattentiveness.

Apart from the burial there was one final duty to perform. I headed to the funeral parlour where Christopher's body was stored. I was to dress him. Christopher lay on a ceramic slab in a small room painted white with lights that were too bright. The funeral director stood behind making encouraging sounds as I struggled to manipulate my brother's corpse. Rigor mortis made the task a welcome and distracting challenge; and when he was clothed in shirt and tie, suit, socks and shoes, I held my brother's hand for the last time.

In the Jamaican culture of my parents' childhood it was the practice of country people to secure the duppies, the spirits of those who, if they had died discontentedly, would roam the earth seeking recompense and revenge on those deemed responsible for their demise. To ensure the duppies would be trapped and could never escape, frightened relatives nailed the shirtsleeves and socks of the recently deceased to the coffin. I looked at Christopher – or more accurately at his corpse. He seemed to be content and in repose. But I was steadily overcome with the feeling that at any minute now Christopher would sit up and drag me down with him, into the coffin. If that was the case, I was determined not to resist. If it was to be so, then so be it. Having failed him in this life it was only right that I should accompany him in the next world. Out of the flood of those thoughts a voice emerged behind me. It was the undertaker. She had been speaking for a while. 'You can let go now,' she said, coaxing me to release my grip from Christopher's hand. 'Just let go.'

Notes

Preface

1 Hughlings Jackson, J., 'On the anatomical, physiological, and pathological investigations of epilepsies', West Riding Lunatic Asylum Medical Report, 1873, 3, pp. 315–49.

2 The aetiology of epilepsy is discussed at length in the first chapter of Gowers's seminal book, *Epilepsy and Other Chronic Convulsive Diseases*.

3 Hughlings Jackson, J., 'On a Particular Variety of Epilepsy ("Intellectual Aura"), One Case with Symptoms of Organic Brain Disease', *Brain*, 1 July 1881.

Just Awake

1 Hunter, W., Introductory Lecture to Students [*c.* 1780], St Thomas's Hospital, MS 55.182.

2 Dostoevsky, F., *The Idiot*, p. 28.

Best Kept Secret

1 Greene, G., *A Sort of Life*, pp. 136–8.

2 Sieveking, E., *On Epilepsy and Epileptiform Seizures*, p. 113.

3 Greene, G., *A Sort of Life*, p. 137.

4 Gowers, W., *Epilepsy and Other Chronic Convulsive Diseases*, p. 8.

5 Author interview, 3 September 2014.

6 Prince John was the sixth and youngest child of George V and Queen Mary. He died aged thirteen in 1919, from a severe epileptic fit.

7 Edward Lear's diaries, 1858–88, are kept at Houghton Library, Harvard College Library, Harvard University, MS Eng. 797.3.

8 Lyndall Gordon's biography of Emily Dickinson, *Lives Like Loaded Guns*, makes a thorough and compelling case for the retrospective diagnosis of the poet's epilepsy, and how it informed her poetry.

9 From Dickinson's poem 'I Felt a Cleaving in my Mind'.

10 From Dickinson's poem 'I Tie my Hat—I Crease my Shawl.'

11 Slater's *Lying* is a strange and unsettling book, a pointedly unreliable memoir which skirts around epilepsy and appears aimed at tying the reader in knots.

12 Tony Greig talks frankly about his epilepsy throughout his 1980 autobiography, *My Story*.

13 In 'No Holds Barred', *Spectator*, 15 September 1978, p. 14, Patrick Marnham gives a round-up of the press's hypocritical reporting on Greig's epilepsy.

14 ONS omnibus survey, November 2001.

Can You Smell Burning?

1 Gershwin's ego was the talk of the town during his lifetime, invariably described by its size – as big as a ballroom. Anna Hamburger was a regular member of Gershwin's retinue.

2 There have been very many misunderstandings and falsehoods advanced over Gershwin's condition. Carp attempted 'to clarify data misconceptions about the illness and pathology' in 'George Gershwin: Illustrious American composer. His fatal glioblastoma', *American Journal of Surgical Pathology* 1979, 3, pp. 473–7. Elena Gasenzer and Edmund Neugebauer give a robust overview in 'George Gershwin: A case of new ways in neurosurgery as well as in the history of Western music', Case Report: History of Neurosurgery, *Acta Neurochirurgica*, June 2014, Vol. 156 (6), pp. 1251–8.

3 Galen's description (394) *De locis affectis*, III, 11, Vol. 8, p. 194, is also recorded in Owsei Temkin's seminal book on epilepsy, *The Falling Sickness*, p. 37.

4 The early descriptions of auras are comprehensively covered by Emmanouil Magiorkinis, Kalliopi Sidiropoulou and Aristidis Diamantis in 'Hallmarks in the History of Epilepsy: From Antiquity till the Twentieth Century', Office for the Study of the History of Hellenic Naval Medicine, Naval Hospital of Athens, Greece.

5 Gowers, W., 'A Clinical Lecture on Minor Epilepsy', *British Medical Journal*, 6 January 1900.

6 Gowers's colleague W. Colman recorded a number of incidences of musical hallucinations amongst his patients in 'Hallucinations in the Sane, Associated with Organic Disease of the Sensory Organs etc.', *British Medical Journal*, 12 May 1894.

7 Critchley, M., 'Musicogenic Epilepsy', *Brain*, 1 March 1937, pp. 13–27.

8 Efron, R., 'The Effect of Olfactory Stimuli in Arresting Uncinate Fits', *Brain*, 1 June 1956, pp. 267–81.

9 Yarmolinsky, A., *Dostoevsky: His Life and Art*.

10 Author interview, 11 January 2014.

11 Badder, D., 'Powell and Pressburger: The War Years', *Sight & Sound*, Winter 1978/9.

12 Powell described his approach to the hallucinations in an interview with *Sight & Sound* in 1978; he explained that he took his cue from a surgeon whom he'd interviewed: 'He uttered another marvellous phrase which really altered the whole conception of the film. He said, "And this illusion can take place in space but not in time." And that's what we showed with the "frozen" Ping-Pong game and David Niven sitting up during the operation with everyone around him frozen in time. There is this whole hallucination taking place in the thousandth of a fraction of a second.'

13 In many instances patients and their friends and relatives have become attuned to their little absences or dreamy states and attribute it to their

character, so that they often present late to the doctor, only once the symptoms become more acute and obvious. In 'Lectures on the Diagnosis of Epilepsy' (*British Medical Journal*, 1 February 1879) Hughlings Jackson reflects that at times the dreamy states are mistaken as mere curiosities.

14 The subject of epilepsy in the film is explored by Diane Broadbent Friedman. Her book *A Matter of Life and Death: The Brain Revealed by the Mind of Michael Powell* is a deconstruction of the neurological condition that ails the pilot.

15 This case was referred to by Sir Charles Symonds at his Hughlings Jackson lecture at the Royal Society of Medicine in March 1959. Symonds explored a number of triggers for the 'excitation and inhibition in epilepsy' including reading and touching.

16 'Prediction of seizure likelihood with a long-term, implanted seizure advisory system in patients with drug-resistant epilepsy: a first-in-man study', *Lancet Neurology*, 2013 June; 12 (6), pp. 563–71.

17 'Neil Young: The *Rolling Stone* Interview', *Rolling Stone*, 9 November 1968. See also Young's *Waging Heavy Peace*.

18 The fallout from Gershwin's death was acrimonious. Accusations were still continuing to fly late into the 1990s when one of his biographers, Edward Jablonski, entered into the fray defending Gershwin's family from a charge of neglect with a letter to the *New York Times* on 25 October 1998 entitled 'George Gershwin: He Couldn't Be Saved'.

The Visitor

1 Vasari, G., *The Lives of the Artists* (part 3).

2 Johann Wolfgang von Goethe, *Italienische Reise*.

3 Friedrich Nietzsche, *Die Geburt de Tragödie*, in Vol. 3/1, *Werke: Kritische Gesamtausgabe*. See also J. Sallis's *Transfigurements: On the True Sense of Art*, p. 9.

4 Honan, W. H., 'Cardiologist Answers a Raphael Question', *New York Times*, 16 December 1995.

5 Dostoevsky, F., *The Idiot*, p. 28.

6 Dostoevsky, A., *Dostoevsky Reminiscences*, p. 18.

7 Dostoevsky, F., *Dostoevsky: Letters and Reminiscences*, p. 54.

8 Dickens, C., *Oliver Twist*, p. 187.

9 Monaco, F. and Mula, M., 'Cesare Lombroso and Epilepsy 100 Years Later: An unabridged report of his original transactions', *Epilepsia*, 52(4), 2011, pp. 679–88.

10 Lombroso, Cesare, *Crime: Its Causes and Remedies*, translated by Henry P. Horton, Little, Brown, 1911.

11 Monaco, F. and Mula, M., 'Cesare Lombroso and Epilepsy 100 Years Later', op. cit.

12 Lombroso's description of Luccheni is transcribed in *Popular Science Monthly*, June 1899. Vincenzo Ruggiero sites the story of Luigi Luccheni and Lombroso in a case study in *Understanding Political Violence: A Criminological Approach*, pp. 44–6.

13 The film is based on the novel *Electricity* by Ray Robinson.

14 Author interview, 6 January 2014.

15 Ibid.

16 Author interview, 15 December 2014.

17 Curtis, I., *So This is Permanence*, Introduction, p. xxii.

18 See Deborah Curtis's foreword to Ian Curtis's *So This is Permanence*.

19 Curtis, I., *So This is Permanence*, Introduction, p. xxiv.

I am Me No More

1 Author interview, 21 January 2014.

2 Dostoevsky, F., *The Idiot*, p. 56.

3 David Thomson in his analysis of *The Big Sleep* (BFI Film Classics), presents a wry take on the Hollywood thriller – a girl with a gun, but the girl is a nymphomaniac prone to petit mal seizures.

4 See *North's Translation of Plutarch's Life of Julius Caesar*, p. 62.

Colonies of Mercy

1 Author interview, 4 December 2014.

2 Dickens, C., *Household Words*. See *The Uncollected Writings of Charles Dickens*.

3 Soon after Bristol, workhouses were established in Worcester, Plymouth, Norwich and Hull.

4 In *History of Madness* Foucault details the policy in numerous European countries of excluding vagrants from city centres. Foucault argues that workhouses and houses of correction followed on from the closure of leper colonies.

5 *New York Times*, 9 November 1902.

6 Steckel, R. and Floud, R., eds, *Health and Welfare during Industrialization*, Introduction and p. 285.

7 'The Colony of Mercy', *Cambridge Tribune*, 20 January 1894.

8 Sellers, E., 'The Story of a Colony for Epileptics', *Popular Science Monthly*, Vol. 42, March 1893.

9 Ibid. Julie Sutter also chronicles the tension between the classes at Bethel.

10 Sutter, J., 'The Colony of Mercy', op. cit.

11 Figures for the rates of mortality in Germany at the end of the nineteenth century are given in 'Heights and Living Standards in Germany, 1850–1939: The Case of Wurttemberg', in Steckel and Floud's *Health and Welfare during Industrialization*, pp. 285–330.

12 Ibid.

13 Sellers, E., 'The Story of a Colony for Epileptics', op. cit.

14 The role of neurologists in the founding of the centre at Chalfont is told in 'The neurological founding fathers of the National Society for Epilepsy and of the Chalfont Centre for Epilepsy' by J.W.A.S. Sander, J. Barclay and S. D. Shorvon. *Journal of Neurology, Neurosurgery, and Psychiatry*, 1993, 56, pp. 599–604.

15 Jean Barclay's *A Caring Community: A centenary history of the National Society for Epilepsy and the Chalfont Centre, 1892–1992*

gives a comprehensive overview of the history of the Chalfont Centre.

16 'London Council's Blight on Epsom', *New York Times*, 17 March 1907. Ewell epileptic colony was one of a cluster of five asylums objected to by Lord Rosebery.

17 *The Times*, 1 February 1895.

18 Barclay, J., *A Caring Community: A Centenary History of the National Society for Epilepsy and the Chalfont Centre, 1892–1992.*

19 Chalfont Centre, Archive, unlabelled box.

20 In 1902 the Committee for a Colony for Epileptics at Warford in Cheshire sent a delegation to the USA to report on conditions at its epileptic colonies. That report, 'Visitor Inspection to Colonies and Hospitals for Epileptics, the Feeble-Minded and the Insane in the USA', by J. Milson Rhodes and Edwin W. Marshall, was published by P. S. King & Son, 1902.

21 *New York Times*, 9 November 1902.

22 'Mr. Townsend Trench. The Healer's Art, A Chat with a Specialist', *Westminster Budget*, 20 December 1895.

23 The eugenicist Albert Priddy served as the first superintendent of the colony. In 1914, Priddy asked permission from the state legislature to expand the colony's remit to include 'the feeble minded'.

24 'What the Work Done in the Eugenics Record Office at Cold Spring Harbour Has Proved in Scientific Race Investigation', *New York Times*, 12 January 1913.

25 Carrie Buck was committed for sterilisation as a seventeen-year-old at Virginia State Colony for Epileptics in Madison Heights near Lynchburg, Virginia.

26 Ben A. Franklin, 'Teenager's Sterilization an Issue Decades Later', *New York Times*, 7 March 1980.

27 Barclay, J., *A Caring Community*, op. cit.

28 Chalfont Centre, Archive, unlabelled box.

29 Author interview, 15 December 2014.

Anger in the Minds of Gods

1 Like many physicians, John Hughlings Jackson worked at numerous hospitals during his career. But he was most closely associated with the London Hospital and the National Hospital for the Relief and Cure of the Paralysed and the Epileptic.

2 Rawlings, B., *A Hospital in the Making: A History of the National Hospital for the Paralysed and Epileptic 1859–1901*, p. 5.

3 Ibid., p. 8.

4 For more background on the use of electricity in Victorian hospitals see Iwan Morus's *Shocking Bodies: Life, Death and Electricity in Victorian England*, p. 148.

5 John Eric Erichsen was a prominent surgeon, president of the Royal College of Surgeons and author of a number of books including *The Science and Art of Surgery*. He made the statement about the limits of brain surgery when addressing an international congress of physicians in London in August 1881.

6 'Sir Victor Horsley's Clinic at the National Hospital for the Paralyzed and Epileptic, Queen Square', *British Journal of Surgery*, Vol. 1, issue 3, 1913, pp. 515–17. See also Fox, Nicholas J., 'Scientific Theory Choice and Social Structure: The Case of Joseph Lister's Antisepsis, Humoral Theory and Asepsis', *History of Science*, Vol. 26, December 1988, pp. 367–397.

7 This remembrance is from Lister's house surgeon, Thompson, in 1883. Thompson, St C., 'Memories of a House Surgeon', *Lancet*, i (1927), pp. 775–80.

8 Horsley, V., 'Brain-Surgery', *British Medical Journal*, Vol. 2, No. 1345 (9 October 1886), pp. 670–75.

9 The trial was widely reported in all the major newspapers of the day and the *BMJ* published a transcript. The background to Ferrier's work was given in detail in a *BMJ* feature later that year. 'Dr. Ferrier's Localisations; For Whose Advantage?', *British Medical Journal*, Vol. 2, No. 1090 (19 November 1881), pp. 822–4.

10 Horsley's observations on the idea of surgery as a last resort were made at the BMA meeting in Toronto in 1906; the dispute between Gowers and Horsley is recounted by Ernest Jones in *Free Associations: Memoirs of a Psychoanalyst*, p. 119.

11 Lyons, J., *The Citizen Surgeon*, p. 118.

12 Ibid., p. 121.

13 BMA conference in Brighton 1886, reported in the *British Medical Journal*, pp. 338–9.

14 Bond, C. J., *Recollections of Student Life and Later Days*, p. 21.

15 Taylor, David C., 'One hundred years of epilepsy surgery: Sir Victor Horsley's contribution', *Journal of Neurology, Neurosurgery and Psychiatry*, 49, 1986, pp. 485–488.

16 Leriche, R., *La Philosophie de la Chirurgie*, Part II, Chapter I.

17 Critchley, M. and E., *John Hughlings Jackson: Father of English Neurology*, p. 37.

18 Ibid., p. 180.

19 Hughlings Jackson, J., 'On a Particular Variety of Epilepsy ("Intellectual Aura"), One Case with Symptoms of Organic Brain Disease', *Brain*, Vol. 11, issue 2, 1 July 1888, pp. 179–207.

20 Taylor and Marsh led the way in uncovering the true identity of Dr Z, aka Arthur T. Myers. Taylor, D. and Marsh, S., 'Hughlings Jackson's Dr Z: The paradigm of temporal lobe epilepsy revealed', *Brain*, Vol. 134, issue 5, 1 May 2011, pp. 1251–1253.

21 Arthur T. Myers's death was reported in *The Times* and the *British Medical Journal*. His epilepsy was only hinted at; never directly expressed.

22 Hughlings Jackson, J. and Colman, W., 'Case of Epilepsy with the Tasting Movements and "Dreamy State"—Very Small Patch of Softening in the Left Uncinate Gyrus', *Brain*, Vol. 21, 1 January 1898, pp. 580–590.

23 By studying epilepsy, neuroscientists were actually investigating the workings of the brain. Hughlings Jackson, J., 'On a Particular Variety

of Epilepsy ("Intellectual Aura"): One Case with Symptoms of Organic Brain Disease', *Brain*, Vol. 11, 1 July 1880, 11, pp. 179–207.

24 'Editorial', *Brain*, Vol. 134, 19 May 2011.

Ticket to Heaven

1 Bible, Mark 9: 17–26.

2 Pliny the Elder, *The Natural History*, translated by Bostock, J. and Riley, T., Book 28, Chapter 7.

3 The Hippocratic approach to epilepsy is outlined in the chapter on 'The Sacred Disease' in *Hippocrates* with an English translation by W.H.S. Jones, pp. 127–184.

4 Herodotus, *The Histories*, Book 3. See also Thomas, R., *Herodotus in Context: Ethnography, Science and the Art of Persuasion*, pp. 333–5 for details on Cambyses' illness.

5 See the chapter on 'The Sacred Disease' in *Hippocrates* with an English translation by W.H.S. Jones.

6 Temkin, O., *The Falling Sickness: A History of Epilepsy from the Greeks to the Beginning of Modern Neurology*, pp. 19–21.

7 Summers, M., ed., *Malleus Maleficarum*, Part II, Question I, Chapter XI. Between 1487 and 1699 the *Malleus Maleficarum* was reprinted more than twenty times.

8 Abu al-Qasim Khalaf ibn 'Abbas az-Zahrawi (AD 936–1013) was also known as Abulcasis.

9 Casaubon, M., *A Treatise Concerning Enthusiasme*. See also Temkin's *The Falling Sickness*, op. cit., pp. 148–9.

10 Gowers, R., *Epilepsy and Other Chronic Convulsive Diseases*, p. 67.

11 Hughlings Jackson, J., 'Lectures on the Diagnosis of Epilepsy', *BMJ*, 1 February 1879.

12 Dostoevsky, F., *Crime and Punishment*, Part IV, Chapter I, p. 277.

13 Penfield, W. and Perot, P., 'The Brain's Record of Auditory and Visual Experience', *Brain*, Vol. 86, Part 4, December 1963, pp. 595–696.

14 Ibid., pp. 601–2.

15 Ibid., pp. 615–7. Six years after the boy's operation the researchers reported that he had been free from seizures, though in that sixth year 'unfortunately he developed paranoid schizophrenia . . . He had shown some evidence of this before the operation although he was perfectly normal at the time of operation.' Eleven years on the medical team were happy to report that the boy was still seizure-free and had 'grown to be a fine young man'.

16 Ibid., pp. 683–93.

17 In 1970 Dewhurst and Beard published a paper that is widely seen as a classic study of the link between religion and epilepsy: Dewhurst, K. and Beard, A., 'Sudden Religious Conversions in Temporal Lobe Epilepsy', *Epilepsy and Behaviour*, Vol. 4, 2003, pp. 78–87. This paper drew on a number of case studies that Beard had conducted with Eliot Slater which they'd published seven years earlier: Slater, E. and Beard, A., 'The Schizophrenia-like Psychoses of Epilepsy. i Psychiatric aspects', *British Journal of Psychiatry*, Vol. 109, issue 458, 1963, pp. 95–112.

18 Maudsley, H., *The Pathology of Mind: A Study of its Distempers, Deformities and Disorders*, p. 446.

19 Fadiman, A., *The Spirit Catches You and You Fall Down: A Hmong Child, Her American Doctors, and the Collision of Two Cultures.*

Bad Brain is Worse than No Brain

1 Ramskill's search for a cure is cited by Simon Shorvon in the essay 'The evolution of epilepsy theory and practice at the National Hospital for the Relief and Cure of Epilepsy, Queen Square, between 1860 and 1910', *Epilepsy and Behaviour*, Vol. 31, February 2014, pp. 228–242. Further details on Ramskill's role in the early days of the National Hospital are found in Holmes, G., *The National Hospital, Queen Square, 1860–1948*. See also *Lancet* (obituary) and Critchley, M., 'The Beginnings of the National Hospital, Queen Square (1859–1860)', *British Medical Journal*, 18 June 1960, 1(5189), pp. 1829–37.

2 Gowers, W., *Epilepsy and Other Chronic Compulsive Diseases*, p. 291.

3 Sieveking, E., *On Epilepsy and Epileptiform Seizures: Their Causes, Pathology, and Treatment*, p. 299.

4 Demaitre, L., *Medieval Medicine: The Art of Healing, from Head to Toe.*

5 Galen, Xɪ, pp. 859f. See also O. Temkin's *The Falling Sickness*, op. cit., p. 25. Recent research has also examined the benefits of peony for people with epilepsy. A study in 1997, 'Protective effects of peony root extract and its components on neuron damage' by T. Tsuda indicated that 'peony root extract and its component, gallotannin, have excellent protective effects on neuron damage in addition to anticonvulsant action by prior oral administration'.

6 Culpeper, N., *Culpeper's English Physician and Complete Herbal*, p. 289.

7 More background on Culpeper is to be found in B. Woolley's admirable *Heal Thyself: Nicholas Culpeper and the Seventeenth-Century Struggle to Bring Medicine to the People.*

8 Turner's Third Morrison Lecture, the Royal College of Physicians of Edinburgh, in 1910.

9 Devinsky, J., 'A diary of epilepsy in the early 1800s', *Epilepsy & Behavior*, Vol. 10, No. 2, 2007, pp. 304–10.

10 Wilks, S., *Lectures on Diseases of the Nervous System*, 1878, p. 320.

11 *Lancet*, 1857, Vol. 69, pp. 527–8.

12 Eadie, M., 'Sir Charles Locock and Potassium Bromide', *Journal of the Royal College of Physicians of Edinburgh*, Vol. 42, issue 3, 2012, pp. 274–279.

13 Temkin, O., *The Falling Sickness*, op. cit, pp. 230–33. See also Duffy, John, 'Masturbation and Clitoridectomy: A Nineteenth-Century View', *Journal of the American Medical Association*, Vol. 86, November 1963, pp. 246–248.

14 Friedlander, W., 'The Rise and Fall of Bromide Therapy in Epilepsy', *Archives in Neurology*, Vol. 57, December 2000.

15 Turner, W., *Epilepsy—A Study of the Idiopathic Disease.* Cited by Shorvon, S., in 'Drug treatment of epilepsy in the century of the

ILAE: The first 50 years, 1909–1958', *Epilepsia*, 50 (Suppl. 3), 2009, pp. 69–92.

16 The quotation of Radcliffe's praise for Locock and his endorsement of Bromide is found in Radcliffe, C., *Lectures on Epilepsy, Pain, Paralysis and Certain Other Disorders of the Nervous Sysytem,* p. 201.

17 Gowers, W., *Epilepsy and Other Chronic Compulsive Diseases,* pp. 252–3.

18 Wilks, S., *Lectures on Diseases of the Nervous System,* 1878, p. 322.

19 Turner, W., op. cit.

20 Clark, L. P., 'A Digest of Recent Work on Epilepsy', *The Journal of Nervous and Mental Disease,* Vol. 27, 1900.

21 Shorvon, S., 'Drug treatment of epilepsy in the century of the ILAE: The first 50 years, 1909–1958', *Epilepsia,* 50 (Suppl. 3), 2009, pp. 69–92.

22 Friedlander, W., 'The Rise and Fall of Bromide Therapy in Epilepsy', *Archives of Neurology* 57, December 2000.

23 Author interview, 8 July 2015.

24 See O. Temkin's *The Falling Sickness,* pp. 234–5 for details on the long history of trepanning.

25 Penfield, W. and Evans, J., 'The Frontal Lobe in Man: A Clinical study of Maximum Removals', *Brain* 1935, 58, pp. 115–33.

26 Penfield, W., *No Man Alone: A Neurosurgeon's Life,* p. 210.

27 *Brain* (2006), 129, pp. 827–29.

28 Penfield, W., *No Man Alone,* op. cit., p. 221.

29 Chenjie, X., 'Understanding the human brain: A lifetime of dedicated pursuit. Interview with Dr. Brenda Milner', *McGill Journal of Medicine,* July 2006, 9 (2), pp. 165–72.

30 Ibid.

31 Scoville, W. and Milner, B., 'Loss of Recent Memory after Bilateral Hippocampal Lesions', *Journal of Neurology, Neurosurgery & Psychiatry,* 1957, 20, p. 11.

32 This concept is explored by D. Penfield and W. Hebb in 'Human Behaviour after Extensive Bilateral Removal from the Frontal Lobes', *Archives of Neurology and Psychiatry* 1940, 44 (2): pp. 421–38.

Persona

1 Sjorbing, H., *Ixophreni. Psykologisk-pedagogisk uppslagsbok*, Stockholm, 1944. Sjorbing's analysis is included in Engel, J. Jr and Pedley, T. A., eds, *Epilepsy: A Comprehensive Textbook,* pp. 342–345.

2 Mitchell, Falconer, Hill, 'Epilepsy with fetishism relieved by temporal lobectomy', *Lancet,* 25 September 1954.

3 Ibid.

4 Geschwind, N., 'Personality Changes in Temporal Lobe Epilepsy', International Classics in Epilepsy and Behaviour: 1974, reproduced in *Epilepsy & Behavior,* 15, 2009, pp. 425–33.

5 Jackson, P. and Lethem,.J., eds, *The Exegesis of Philip K. Dick.* pp. 36–7.

6 Gopnik, A., 'Blows Against the Empire', *New Yorker,* 20 August 2007.

7 Jackson, P. and Lethem, J., eds, op. cit., Introduction p. xx.

8 Ibid., p. 21.

9 Geschwind, N., 'Personality Changes in Temporal Lobe Epilepsy', op. cit., pp. 425–33.

10 Cited by LaPlante, E., in 'The Riddle of TLE', *Atlantic Monthly,* November 1988.

11 Alajouanine, T., 'Dostoiewski's Epilepsy', *Brain,* Vol. 86, Part 2, pp. 209–18.

12 Ibid.

13 Jackson, P. and Lethem, J., eds, op cit., p. 658.

14 Hesdorffer, D. et al, 'Depression and suicide attempt as risk factors for incident unprovoked seizures', *Annals of Neurology,* 59, 2006, pp. 35–41.

15 Devinsky, J. and Schachter, S., 'Norman Geschwind's contribution to the understanding of behavioural changes in temporal lobe epilepsy': The February 1974 lecture, *Epilepsy & Behavior,* Vol. 15, issue 4, August 2009, pp. 417–24.

16 Hughes, J., 'A reappraisal of the possible seizures of Vincent Van Gogh', *Epilepsy & Behavior,* Vol. 6, 2005, pp. 504–10.

17 Jansen, L., Luijten, H. and Bakker, N., *Vincent Van Gogh: The Letters*. Fabienne Picard felicitously analysed the letters in a letter to the editor, *Epilepsy & Behavior*, Vol. 22, 2011, pp. 414–15.

18 'V. S. Ramachandran: Sharpening Up "The Science of Art". An Interview with Anthony Freeman', *Journal of Consciousness Studies*, 8, No. 1, 2001, pp. 9–29. See also Ramachandran, V. S. and Hirstein, W., 'The Science of Art: A Neurological Theory of Aesthetic Experience', *Journal of Consciousness Studies*, 6, No. 6–7, 1999, pp. 15–51.

19 Historical figures such as Napoleon have been at the centre of this debate. J. Hughes offers a snapshot of the perils of retrospective diagnosis in: 'Did all those famous people really have epilepsy?', *Epilepsy & Behavior*, Vol. 6, issue 2, March 2005, pp. 115–39.

20 Thomas, R., 'Epilepsy: creative sparks', *Practical Neurology*, 2010, 10, pp. 219–26.

21 Jansen, L., Luijten, H. and Bakker, N., *Vincent Van Gogh: The Letters*, op cit.

Grand Mal

1 'De novo mutations in epileptic encephalopathies', *Nature*, 501, pp. 217–21, 12 September 2013. See also 'Largest study of epilepsy patients ever conducted reveals new and surprising genetic risk factors', *EurekAlert*, 12 August 2013.

2 Author interview, 16 August 2015.

3 Spratling, W., *Epilepsy and its Treatment*. SUDEP is defined as sudden, unexpected, witnessed or unwitnessed, non-traumatic and non-drowning death in patients with epilepsy, with or without evidence of a seizure and excluding documented *status epilepticus*, in which post-mortem examination does not reveal a toxicological or anatomical cause of death.

Acknowledgements

It has been heartening to be able to work again with Dan Franklin and the team at Jonathan Cape in bringing this book to life. I tip my hat at my friend and agent Sophie Lambert and her colleagues at Conville & Walsh who have nurtured me and the writing of *A Smell of Burning*.

I am especially grateful to the many people whom I interviewed for the book and to the members of Epilepsy Society who have supported this project, loaned books to me and opened up their archives.

It has been my ambition to give a human face to epilepsy, and to conjure my brother in these pages. If family and friends have managed to read this far, then I hope they will at least recognise that ambition.

I would very much like to thank my brother, Christopher.

Bibliography

Barclay, Jean, *A Caring Community: A Centenary History of the National Society for Epilepsy and the Chalfont Centre, 1892–1992*. National Society for Epilepsy, 1992.

Bond, C. J., *Recollections of Student Life and Later Days*. H. K. Lewis & Co., 1939.

Casaubon, Meric, *A Treatise Concerning Enthusiasme* (1655). Scholars' Facsimiles & Reprints, 1970.

Christie, Ian, *A Matter of Life and Death*. British Film Institute, 2000.

Corkin, Suzanne, *Permanent Present Tense: The Unforgettable Life of the Amnesic Patient, H.M.* Basic Books, 2013.

Critchley, Macdonald and Eileen, *John Hughlings Jackson: Father of English Neurology*. Oxford University Press, 1998.

Culpeper, Nicholas, *Culpeper's English Physician and Complete Herbal*. J. Scatcherd, 1801.

Curtis, Ian, eds Deborah Curtis and Jon Savage, *So This is Permanence: Joy Division Lyrics and Notebooks*. Faber & Faber, 2014.

Demaitre, Luke, *Medieval Medicine: The Art of Healing, from Head to Toe*. Praeger, 2013.

Dick, Philip K., eds Pamela Jackson and Jonathan Lethem, *The Exegesis of Philip K. Dick*. Gollancz 2011.

Dickens, Charles, *Oliver Twist*. Penguin Classics, 2007.

Dickens, Charles, ed. Harry Stone, *The Uncollected Writings of Charles Dickens: 'Household Words', 1850–1859*. Allen Lane, 1969.

Dickinson, Emily, ed. Thomas H. Johnson, *The Complete Poems*. Faber & Faber, 1976.

Dostoevsky, Anna, translated by Beatrice Stillman, *Dostoevsky Reminiscences*. Wildwood House, 1976.

Dostoevsky, Fyodor, translated by Constance Garnett, *Crime and Punishment*. Wordsworth Editions, 2000.

Dostoevsky, Fyodor, translated by David Magarshack, *The Idiot*. Penguin Books, 1955.

Dostoevsky, Fyodor, translated by S. S. Koteliansky and J. Middleton Murray, *Dostoevsky: Letters and Reminiscences*. Chatto & Windus, 1923.

Engel, Jerome Jr and Pedley, Timothy A., eds, *Epilepsy: A Comprehensive Textbook*. Lippincott Williams & Wilkins, 2007.

Erichsen, John Eric, *The Science and Art of Surgery*. Longmans, Green, 1877.

Evans, Margiad, *A Ray of Darkness*. John Calder, 1978.

Fadiman, Anne, *The Spirit Catches You and You Fall Down: A Hmong Child, Her American Doctors, and the Collision of Two Cultures*. Farrar, Straus and Giroux, 1999.

Foucault, Michel, ed. Jean Khalfa, translated by Jonathan Murphy, *History of Madness*. Routledge, 2006.

Friedman, Diane Broadbent, *A Matter of Life and Death: The Brain Revealed by the Mind of Michael Powell*. AuthorHouse, 2008.

Galen, eds Kraus, Paulus and Walzer, Richardus, *Compendium Timaei Platoni*. Warburg Institute, 1951.

Gordon, Lyndall, *Lives Like Loaded Guns, Emily Dickinson and Her Family's Feuds*. Virago, 2010.

Gowers, William Richard, *Epilepsy and other Chronic Convulsive Diseases*. J. & A. Churchill, 1881.

Greene, Graham, *A Sort of Life*. Penguin, 1993.

Greig, Tony, *My Story*. Hutchinson, 1980.

Herodotus, translated by G. Woodrouffe Harris, *The Histories*. 1906.

Hippocrates, translated by W.H.S. Jones, *Hippocrates*. Loeb, 1923–31.

Holmes, Gordon, *The National Hospital, Queen Square, 1860–1948*. E. & S. Livingstone, 1954.

Jablonski, Edward, *Gershwin*. De Capo Press, 1988.

Jackson, Pamela and Lethem, Jonathan, eds, *The Exegesis of Philip K. Dick*. Gollancz, 2011.

Jansen, Leo, Luijten, Hans and Bakker, Nienke, eds, *Vincent Van Gogh: The Letters: The Complete Illustrated and Annotated Edition (Vol.1–6)*. Thames & Hudson, 2009.

Jones, Ernest, *Free Associations: Memoirs of a Psychoanalyst*. Basic Books, 1959.

Kramer, Heinrich and Sprenger, James, translated by the Reverend Montague Summers, *Malleus Maleficarum*. Dover Publications, 1978.

Leriche, René, *La Philosophie de La Chirurgie*. Flammarion, 1951.

Lombroso, Cesare, *Crime: Its Causes and Remedies*, translated by Henry P. Horton. Little, Brown, 1911.

Lyons, John Benignus, *The Citizen Surgeon: A Biography of Sir Victor Horsley, 1857–1916*. Peter Dawnay, 1966.

Maudsley, Henry, *The Pathology of Mind: A Study of its Distempers, Deformities, and Disorders*. Macmillan & Co., 1895.

Morus, Iwan, *Shocking Bodies: Life, Death and Electricity in Victorian England*. The History Press, 2011.

Noakes, Vivien, *Edward Lear: The Life of a Wanderer*. The History Press, 2006.

Penfield, Wilder, *No Man Alone: A Neurosurgeon's Life*. Little, Brown, 1977.

Pliny the Elder, *The Natural History*, translated by Bostock, John and Riley, Thomas Taylor and Francis, 1855.

Plutarch, *North's Translation of Plutarch's Life of Julius Caesar*. BiblioLife, 2015.

Radcliffe, Charles Bland, *Lectures on Epilepsy, Pain, Paralysis and Certain Other Disorders of the Nervous System*. Lindsay and Blakiston, 1866.

Rawlings, B. Buford, *A Hospital in the Making: A History of the National Hospital for the Paralysed and Epileptic (Albany Memorial) 1859–1901*. Sir Isaac Pitman & Sons, 1913.

Robinson, Ray, *Electricity*. Black Cat, 2006.

Sacks, Oliver, *Hallucinations*. Picador, 2012.

Sallis, John, *Transfigurements: On the True Sense of Art*. University of Chicago Press, 2011.

Sieveking, Sir Edward Henry, *On Epilepsy and Epileptiform Seizures: Their Causes, Pathology, and Treatment*. John Churchill, 1858.

Slater, Lauren, *Lying: A Metaphorical Memoir*. Penguin Books, 2001.

Spratling, William, *Epilepsy and its Treatment*. W. B. Saunders & Co., 1904.

Steckel, Richard H. and Floud, Roderick, eds, *Health and Welfare during Industrialization*. University of Chicago Press, 1997.

Sutter, Julie, *A Colony of Mercy, or, Social Christianity at Work, etc. A description of a home for epileptics at Bethel, near Bielefeld*. Hodder & Stoughton, 1893.

Temkin, Owsei, *The Falling Sickness: A History of Epilepsy from the Greeks to the Beginnings of Modern Neurology*. The Johns Hopkins Press, 1971.

Thomson, David, *The Big Sleep*. British Film Institute, 1997.

Tossell, David, *Tony Greig: A Reappraisal of English Cricket's Most Controversial Captain*. Pitch, 1988.

Vasari, Giorgio, translated by Julia Conway Bondanella and Peter Bondanella, *The Lives of the Artists*. Oxford University Press, 2008.

Wilks, Sir Samuel, *Lectures on Diseases of the Nervous System: Delivered at Guys Hospital*. J&A Churchill, 1878.

Woolley, Benjamin, *Heal Thyself: Nicholas Culpeper and the Seventeenth-Century Struggle to Bring Medicine to the People*. HarperCollins Publishers, 2004.

Yarmolinsky, Avrahm, *Dostoevsky: His Life and Art*. S. G. Phillips, Inc., 1957.

Young, Neil, *Waging Heavy Peace: A Hippy Dream*. Viking, 2012.

Index

Index

Fadiman, Anne 156
Falconer and James 44
Falling Sickness 79
Farncombe, Anne 94
Ferrier, David 117, 118, 119, 128
First World War 105, 106, 173–4
focal motor seizures 125
Foerster, Otfrid 179
Foucault, Michel 222
Freud, Sigmund 132, 148–9

Gachet, Dr 200
Galen 30–32, 164
Galton, Francis 106
genetics, gene therapy 208–9
George V 19, 85
Gershwin, George 29–30, 40, 46, 218, 220
Geschwind, Norman 192–3, 198
Geschwind's syndrome 193, 195, 197, 200, 201
Gopnik, Adam 196
Gordon, Lyndall 20
Goulstonian lectures (1860) 163
Gowers, William 12, 32, 33, 36, 117, 119–20, 145, 146, 163, 170, 194, 224
grand mal epilepsy 8, 70, 189
Grannie Reid 47–50
Grant, Christopher
  after-effects of seizures 53
  approach to his condition 22, 23, 68, 156–7
  becomes an altar boy 16–18
  bizarre behaviour of 161–2, 188
  church's intervention 135–6
  death of 211–15
  diagnosed as epileptic 10–11, 111
  ecstatic state 160
  effect of epilepsy on his temperament 190
  fainting incidents 8, 9, 10, 16, 18, 33

father's attitude towards 28
hospital misdiagnosis of 111–14
love of cars 73–6
makes film 203
mother's attitude towards 9–11, 33, 72–5, 162
requests bagpipes at his funeral 189–90
timing of onset of seizures 43
Grant, Sonia 211–12, 213
Greene, Graham 11–13
Greig, Tony 24–8
Gutsell, Pat 107

hallucinations/visions 41, 140–46, 152–9, 219
Hauptmann, Alfred 173
Herodotus 137–8
Hindu Marriage Act (1955) 13
Hippocrates 138
The Histories (Herodotus) 137–8
history-taking 1, 2–4, 112, 123
Hitler, Adolf 106
H.M. *see* Molaison, Henry Gustav
Hmong people 156
Hogarth, William 110
Holbein, Hans 55–6
Hôpital Général, Paris 87
Horsley, Siward 122–3, 125
Horsley, Victor Alexander 115–23, 125, 225
Hughlings Jackson, John 37–8, 42, 108, 114, 118, 123–32, 145, 146, 150, 194, 200, 224
Hunter, William 2
hysterical epilepsy 169

The Idiot (Dostoevsky) 6, 53–6, 67–8, 71, 147, 198
India, Indians 13–15
insula 154–6

239

A Smell of Burning